_In_　　　　　　　　　　　　　　MW01291729

Praise for the authors' previous best-selling book,
Extended Massive Orgasm

"They are breaking new ground—and, who knows,
maybe Guinness world records, too—in orgasmic studies."
San Francisco Chronicle

"It covers everything imaginable to do with 'clitorology,' as they call it.
It's easy to understand and written without frills, in correct
and graphic language, with chapters on everything to do
with the whole sex package, including male orgasm."
The Sunday Times Magazine

"Check chapter 5 for the most detailed directions
to the G-spot we've ever seen."
_GQ_

"The book's detailed instructions cover how to lubricate
your honey's sweet spot, how to 'anchor' the clitoris to keep it
from slipping away from you, how to properly 'stroke' the clitoris
with your fingers, using different speeds and motions, and
what to do with your nonstroking hand."
Playboy.com

"What man doesn't want to please the gals? Who doesn't want
more pleasure? Bodansky's book can help here
and has the added joy of being funny at times...."
The Espresso

Other titles in the Positively Sexual series

Ordering

Trade bookstores in the U.S. and Canada please contact:

Publishers Group West
1700 Fourth Street, Berkeley CA 94710
Phone: (800) 788-3123   Fax: (800) 351-5073

Hunter House books are available at bulk discounts for textbook course adoptions; to qualifying community, health-care, and government organizations; and for special promotions and fund-raising.
For details please contact:

Special Sales Department
Hunter House Inc., PO Box 2914, Alameda CA 94501-0914
Phone: (510) 865-5282   Fax: (510) 865-4295
E-mail: ordering@hunterhouse.com

Individuals can order our books from most bookstores, by calling **(800) 266-5592**, or from our website at **www.hunterhouse.com**

✦ *Instant Orgasm* ✦

Excitement at First Touch!

Steve Bodansky, PhD

&

Vera Bodansky, PhD

Hunter House Inc., Publishers
PO Box 2914
Alameda CA 94501-0914

Library of Congress Cataloging-in-Publication Data
Bodansky, Steve.
    Instant orgasm : excitement at first touch! / Steve Bodansky and Vera Bodansky. — 1st ed.
        p. cm. — (Positively sexual)
    Includes bibliographical references and index.
    ISBN-13: 978-0-89793-508-1 (pbk.)
    ISBN-10: 0-89793-508-X (pbk.)
    1. Sexual excitement.   2. Orgasm.   3. Sex instruction.   I. Bodansky, Vera.   II. Title.
HQ31.B59333 2008
613.9'6—dc22   2007048896

Project Credits

Cover Design: Brian Dittmar
  Graphic Design
Book Production: John McKercher
Developmental and Copy Editor:
  Kelley Blewster
Proofreader: John David Marion
Indexer: Nancy D. Peterson
Acquisitions Editor: Jeanne Brondino
Editor: Alexandra Mummery

Senior Marketing Associate: Reina Santana
Publicity Assistant: Alexi Ueltzen
Rights Coordinator: Candace Groskreutz
Customer Service Manager:
  Christina Sverdrup
Order Fulfillment: Washul Lakdhon
Administrator: Theresa Nelson
Computer Support: Peter Eichelberger
Publisher: Kiran S. Rana

Printed and Bound by Bang Printing, Brainerd, Minnesota

Manufactured in the United States of America

9 8 7 6 5 4 3 2 1   First Edition   08 09 10 11 12

Contents

Chapter 3
PLEASURE TRAINING

Chapter 4
PARTNERED PLEASURE

⇒ Important Note ⇐

The material in this book is intended to provide a review of information regarding sexual techniques. Every effort has been made to provide accurate and dependable information. We believe that the sensuality advice given in this book poses no risk to any healthy person. However, if you have any sexually transmitted diseases, we recommend consulting your doctor before using this book.

The publisher, authors, and editors, as well as the professionals quoted in the book, cannot be held responsible for any error, omission, professional disagreement, or dated material, and are not liable for any damage, injury, or other adverse outcome of applying any of the information resources cited in this book. If you have questions concerning the application of the information described in this book, consult a qualified professional.

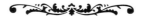

List of Illustrations

Acknowledgments

We wonder if most people even read the Acknowledgments. It does not matter. Acknowledging is mainly for those who are doing it. Of course, it is nice to receive someone's "thank you," but the one who benefits the most is the acknowledger.

We asked the publisher for our previous editor, Kelley Blewster, and are so pleased that she said yes. She takes our original streams of consciousness and makes them into precise and concise thoughts that hit their mark. She deserves just as much credit as we do for this book.

We really appreciate Regena Thomashauer for her continued love and support, and also for all of her "Sister Goddesses" who have donated their bodies for the cause. Many of the questions that we have addressed have come from them. We think that a person learns best from teaching, and we are so fortunate to be able to serve real desire in our capacity as teachers. We would also like to thank Dame Lori Sutherland for her kindness and support in sending desirous women to see us, and also for her own special desires.

We are thankful to the people at Hunter House Publishers, who have stuck by us enthusiastically through the years, including Kiran Rana, Jeanne Brondino, Alex Mummery, and Christina Sverdrup.

We have not forgotten how we got here and are continually indebted to our training at the hands of Vic and Cindy Baranco and the gang at Morehouse.

We would also like to thank illustrators Teri Sugg, Kim Black, and the folks at paintyourlife.com, who came through like champs.

We would like to express a sincere and loving appreciation to Bruce Thomashauer for his friendship and the scintillating ideas he shared with us over the phone.

I (Steve) am grateful to Dr. Loosli, who gave me exercises for my frozen shoulder, and to Clair Davies, author of *The Trigger Point Therapy Workbook,* which reliably keeps the pain away. A bright smile to Dr. Cliff Broshinsky, who worked on my painful gums and teeth and made them feel the best they have in years.

And, dear readers, we are most thankful to you for your appreciation of our works.

Some Definitions to Know Up Front

There are a number of terms used throughout this book that come from our earlier works and that you, the reader, should be made familiar with right from the start:

EMO (extended massive orgasm): An orgasm of great intensity that lasts for a long time—several minutes or even possibly hours.

IO (instant orgasm): A woman's ability to feel orgasmic by focusing her attention on the pleasure of her clitoris on or before the first touch.

peak (*n*): The highest point reached in each cycle of an orgasm. As in a mountain range, there can be many peaks in an orgasm.

to peak (*v*): To notice when the highest point of the orgasmic cycle is reached and to deliberately reduce the orgasm's intensity by stopping or changing the stroke. From here, the giver of the orgasm can intentionally continue the orgasm by creating more intensity, progressing toward another peak.

turn-on: When a woman is in agreement with her desires, either sexual or otherwise, and can stimulate a response in her own or another person's body to gratify those desires.

tumescence: Derived from the Latin word tumor, which means "to swell" or "to engorge." We use the term to indicate an increase in sexual energy, or, during an orgasm, an intensification of the energy that drives the orgasm. It is synonymous with the phrase "going up."

detumescence: A decrease in sexual energy. In an orgasm, the term refers to the waning of physical intensity. It is synonymous with the phrase "coming down."

A Touch of Heaven

It seems like only yesterday that we met,
yet you look better now than you did then,
and then you were a ten.

Many years we have spent together and it still feels pure,
it still feels grand; there is still that same amour and even more.

I wake up and you are sleeping quietly, sweetly.
I kiss your cheek and you stir so neatly. I speak your name
and you are ready to play; maybe first just coffee
and you will give me my way.

During the day I can see paradise in every scene,
utopia in each step, and bliss with each breath.

There is no turning back, which is fine when you are there at my side;
viewing you and the viewpoints you define make it wonderful to go on.

To touch you is to feel heaven, to experience ecstasy,
to capture rapture in your magnificent texture.

The days may get on; perhaps we get older,
yet our love becomes stronger and lovelier and more encompassing.

You are and always will be my dear sweet Valentine.

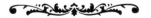

DEDICATION

This book is dedicated to those who have been trailblazers
on the journey toward pleasure, specifically Dr. Vic Baranco.
It is also dedicated to those who have chosen this path.

Introduction

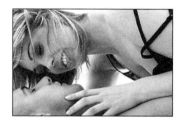

*E*very journey begins with the first step. This book spotlights that first step over and over. If you decide to read this book you will be going on many journeys. There will be trips, rides, and expeditions to an abundance of pleasure. You will get to where you are going by enjoying the path.

We have named this book Instant Orgasm *because we want to focus your attention on our human potential and on what is sensually possible, and we want to build on what we have covered in our previous books on extended massive orgasm. However, the title may be a little misleading for a couple of reasons. First of all, it would probably be more*

more precise to call it *Instantly Orgasmic.* We are not saying that the orgasm lasts for an instant but rather that a person can become orgasmic in an instant. This instant can be extended for however long one desires, one stroke at a time. The second issue is that this ability to be instantly orgasmic exists in women and not in men, although men's ability to feel pleasure instantly can be dramatically improved, too.

Pleasure is always available just around the next corner—but are you having pleasure right now? You can. Orgasm is cost effective. Instant orgasm will cost you something to get, but the results will be well worth your while. You can have it whenever you desire. The price is only some attention, time, and practice. As we have just stated, this is especially true for women and less true for men, although they, too, can have way more immediate pleasure than they currently do. That is what this book is about: how to invest a little time and attention in creating an orgasmic experience whenever you choose. We will give you specific ways to experience this natural phenomenon while still functioning in society. Do not worry that you will become some nonfunctioning, tripped-out hedonist. Your positive influence on your friends and associates and on the world in general will actually increase. The caveat is that you will have to read this book; merely putting it under your pillow and hoping for results will not suffice. And furthermore you will have to practice the techniques regularly, especially at first. To get the most out of this work you will have to rearrange your priorities to place pleasure at the top of the list, at least for a while. You may learn that once you make pleasure a priority your other concerns will all be appropriately addressed. Your life will actually make more sense. You can always rearrange your priorities later if this does not work out, though we doubt that you will want to.

➣ How This Book Works ➣

In this book we describe many times how to pleasure one's partner, focusing on different details with each approach. While we therefore end up repeating certain information, each time we add a new twist or additional information that will add to your understanding of just how to receive and give pleasure. Each sensual or sexual act can be seen as merely a repetitive experience with the same old person, or it can be viewed as an entirely new experience that you enter with an open mind and a novel and fresh approach.

In our earlier books we deliberately took the reader on a mental trip through an orgasm, from beginning to end. We started by describing pleasure, slowly took you higher, peaked you, and then intentionally brought you down. In this book we constantly give you opportunities to feel each "stroke," if you will, one at a time, continually taking you up and down on short orgasmic rides. There is no exact high point, and there is no nice and tidy finish. The pleasure of being instantly orgasmic can happen on any page, including this one. All you have to do is put your attention on your genitals. If you are unable to create this experience at this time, hopefully before you finish reading the book that will change. If you are able to, congratulations! We are confident that we can take you even higher.

Although in different parts of this book we write about similar acts, we place emphasis on different aspects of the experience. For example, in both the "Pleasure Training" chapter and the "Partnered Pleasure" chapter we describe how to rub on a woman's clitoris. In the chapter on training we stress the importance of a couple's verbal exchanges regarding the experience, while in the chapter on pleasuring we emphasize the position of the "pleasure giver's" hands, and we pay more detailed attention to specific strokes. At other times we discuss *both* communication skills and actual techniques, such as in the chapters "Advanced Tips for Creating Orgasms" and "The Pleasure of Peaking." By combining the information in all these chapters and reading the material on self-pleasuring—even the information about self-pleasuring that is addressed to the opposite sex—we believe that a reader can obtain a well-rounded education on pleasuring one's partner and expanding one's own orgasm.

It is fine to practice the techniques described in any chapter of this book immediately after reading the chapter; we even recommend it. However, we also recommend studying the entire book before expecting to be able to apply the information with any skill. If one is knowledgeable about the techniques but lacks communication skills, then obviously one must spend more time reading and rereading the material on communication. It is important to master all the parts of both giving and receiving pleasure if one wishes to become a class-A sexer. In order to become great at receiving orgasms, it will help if you have also learned how to give them. Likewise, the better you are at receiving pleasure, the better you will be at giving it.

Another difference between this book and our earlier books is that in this one we have located the information about men close to similar information about women, rather than dividing chapters up along gender lines. On occasion we describe some differences between the sexes, but for the most part we are speaking to both sexes at once. Again, we think you will get the most out of this book if you read all of it, even those parts relating to the other sex, as it contains a wealth of information that will make you a better lover no matter what sex you are.

We have included information about pleasuring and about ways of being pleasured that we did not cover fully in our other books; that is, in addition to the emphasis on instant orgasm, we have incorporated more details about giving and receiving extended massive orgasms (EMOs). The ability to give an EMO takes practice. Learning more ideas and techniques for doing so will produce a reservoir of knowledge that a person can tap into to be more inventive in creating extended massive fun in bed.

It is essential that fun remain the overriding goal of any sensual encounter, whether it takes place with one's lover or with oneself. This book covers a lot of information, yet we believe that someone who knows little or nothing about sensuality can catch on quickly. There is plenty of useful information for the expert, too.

We conclude the book with our answers to some questions that we have received since our last book.

≽ "No Time" and Other Excuses ≼

When we wrote and talked about extended massive orgasm, one of the usual comments we heard was "When do you think we would have time to do that?" We would explain that, yes, we were talking about extended orgasms, but, no, they do not all have to last for an hour or longer. We pointed out that the major reason we demonstrated hour-long orgasms was to show that they were possible, yet we did not really expect most people to repeatedly try to do what we were doing. One of the main things we wanted to convey about an extended massive orgasm is that people have the ability to begin orgasming on the first stroke or even before. Beyond that, even if you did it for "only" five minutes you would still be having a five-minute orgasm, which is way more than most people allow themselves. Somehow this point got lost in the idea of doing it for hours and hours. In this book we want to emphasize that coming from the very beginning is not only possible (for women) but also easily achieved. (Yes, increasing the intensity of this initial moment will take practice and disciplined—fun—dedication.) We are hereby removing the "no time" excuse from your bag of resistances. All you require is a second. Now you will have to dig into your bag and find some new excuse.

Another resistance we encounter is the belief that studying and learning and practicing will somehow limit a person's creativity. That is just lazy thinking. We knew a beautiful young woman who met a potential lover. He said he was interested in becoming the "world's best lover." She thought this could be great because he was also cute. She told him about her sensual studies and offered to show him our book. He said that he did not want to read from another man's point of view as it would cramp his style. Needless to say, he never got to show her his stuff as he really did not want to learn and she wanted someone who was more open-minded.

⋙ Pleasure Now ⋘

For most people, the ability to feel instant orgasmic pleasure is there. But most of us are so conditioned into thinking that it takes a certain amount of time to reach orgasm that we do not believe there is a simpler way to do it. And even if we know that it takes just a moment of our focused attention to have an orgasm, we still don't let ourselves do it because we believe we have more important things to do or that we do not deserve such pleasure. We have all received messages from our society that say pleasure is sinful, and thus to sin on a whim must be doubly sinful. Furthermore, our minds are filled with thoughts, many of which are negative, about guilt and about defending who we are and justifying ourselves. They are also filled with everyday business and tedious, habitual clutter. There is little availability to attend to pleasure, unless one is deliberate about it. If you intentionally create space and time in your mind for pleasure, you will be surprised by how easy it is to do it and how the negative thoughts and clutter will vanish, at least temporarily.

Let us use our experience as writers to illustrate what we mean. In order for us to teach and write about pleasure it is important for us to act in as pleasurable a way as possible. Therefore, it wouldn't make sense for us to labor for endless hours over a book manuscript, neglecting other parts of our lives, to the point where all pleasure was lost. It might even be hypocritical. So how will we accomplish the demanding task of writing a book while enjoying the process? Will we only write when we feel like it, when it feels right, when it is fun to do so? Writing requires some discipline, so waiting until the good feelings just happen to show up and overwhelm us may not be an honest approach either. Writing and many other endeavors are comparable to having sex in that sometimes you may not have a great desire or a chemical urge to do so, yet once you sit down at the keyboard and start typing, or once you start touching yourself or your partner, the juices start flowing and the desire is created—instantly at times. Therefore, we claim the middle ground, which is to work on this book with as much dedication as we can muster while still enjoying every minute.

While writing this book I had a couple of minor medical problems that kept me away from the keyboard. My shoulder froze up, which could have been caused by repetitive motions such as typing (or stroking clitorises?)—the cause was unknown. But I stayed away from writing and also from repetitive sensual movements (you can overdo anything) for a couple of months, and now that I am feeling better I type for only thirty to sixty minutes at a time, and usually just once or twice a day. I also had a problem with dry eyes; my eyes function better if I do not spend long hours staring at the computer monitor. Taking it slowly gave Vera and me more time to discuss the issues in the book and to make up for lost time in bed. I have found that ignoring my body and sitting for a long time at the computer to meet a writing deadline is counterproductive because it causes my back to hurt so intensely that I must take a break for the following few days. I have gotten better at pacing myself so that writing has become a more and more pleasurable activity.

We have found that this approach to life has enabled us to live an existence that we thoroughly enjoy and wish to continue enjoying. We like to think that we practice what we preach. As we tell our students about sensual experiences, "Taking breaks is beneficial and helpful in creating more pleasure." Likewise, when reading this book, it may be a good idea for you to take a break on occasion. Do not try to read everything at once; instead, try out some of the information and techniques we present before reading more. In addition, practice simply putting your attention on pleasure for brief moments throughout the day. Then you can read further and gain additional skill.

~

As in our other books, we usually use the proper terms for sexual organs and the sexual act; however, we sometimes use the more racy terms when doing so seems appropriate. We have found that most people do not mind those "vulgar" words, and many actually prefer them, but to those of you who may be offended by them we apologize in advance.

When referring to ourselves, we sometimes use "we" and at other times "I." The "we" is, of course, Vera and Steve, and the "I" is just Steve. It is my voice, Steve's, that you are listening to, but it is Vera's voice that I listen to.

CHAPTER 1

Opening Your Mind

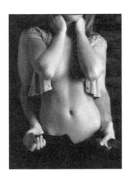

*W*e believe that women have the ability to experience instant orgasmic sensation because they are the source of turn-on. By this we mean that in mammals it is the female that goes into heat and the male that responds. Female humans have an added ability to turn on at will, not just when their menstrual cycle dictates. Because female humans can turn on at will, by putting their full attention on their pleasure area— on their pussy, as we like to say—they can experience all the pleasure that is available. Their genitals can get wet, throb, and feel so much pleasure that we have no problem calling this an orgasm. The more a woman can approve of these wonderful sensations, the better the orgasm will be.

We have coached many women students over the years. Most are not able to easily feel that first stroke on an erogenous zone when they first start out, nor are they fully able to feel their genitals by just focusing their attention on them. Yet, with practice, they have all learned to feel much more than they did before their training, and most become able to experience quite a bit of intense orgasmic sensation with that first eagerly anticipated stroke. The touch does not even have to be directly on their clitoris; it can be almost anywhere on their genitals or on a body part that they have learned to "connect" to their clitoris. (For more on connecting different body parts, see Chapter 2, "Self-Pleasure.") Practice makes it easier to feel the pleasure and causes the initial sensation to intensify dramatically.

The more one practices and grows familiar with her instantly orgasmic potential, the greater becomes her ability to experience an instantly massive or intense orgasm. When Vera began doing orgasm demonstrations, her coach told her to initially hold back to avoid scaring students off. The goal was to gradually build on the orgasm. However, we have taught a number of women to experience this level of intensity immediately, which shows that it is possible to have a "massive" orgasm from the get-go.

In order for women to have an instant orgasm they do not have to do anything other than focus their attention, feel the sensations, and approve of (that is, appreciate) what they're feeling. These three actions are also the road to extending and intensifying the experience. Once a woman has a partner who begins to actively assist in her pleasure production, she only has to continue to do these three things—that is, to focus, feel, and approve—and, of course, to stay relaxed. She will also have to train her partner. (We've included an entire chapter on training techniques.) But even when doing it to yourself, focusing, feeling, and approving are how you increase your pleasure. We will discuss approval in greater detail in the chapter "Partnered Pleasure."

Many people, both men and women, think they have to do more than feel and approve when they are receiving an orgasm. They think they have to assist in the production of the pleasure by moving—by thrusting their hips and tensing up. This straining is actually counterproductive to feeling pleasure. Just understanding the words "tensing" and "straining" should be a clue that they won't take you in the direction of pleasure. Pleasure is about enjoying the experience. More precisely, it is about fully experiencing the moment. When a person is in solely a "helping out" mode, they are not experiencing as much pleasure as they might.

⇒ Give Your Hands a Hand ⇐

We would like to clarify here that the major part of our research, and therefore the focus of the information we present to you, is based on hands-to-genital stimulation. Humans' hands are masterful and dexterous and can perform for a long period of time without getting tired or, unlike genitals, having to be engorged. They provide the best, most efficient way of producing pleasure in a human's body. While using the hands may not be seen as the most erotic or the most intimate way to give pleasure, we could argue that point, too.

Still, even during oral sex it is important for the person receiving the pleasure to relax their body and avoid moving around in response to the stimulus. Intercourse is different; some movement is vital to the act, although probably less and definitely slower than most people realize. A woman's ability to feel more before the first touch, merely through anticipation, as well as her capacity for instant orgasm, can be enhanced with any sex act, including intercourse. She will no longer have to merely lie there and wait for it to happen. A woman's ability to orgasm on the first stroke can also be beneficial to men who worry about premature ejaculation, a subject we hear about from a lot of guys. The man who learns these skills will no longer have to worry about his performance. He can relax, confident that his partner will already be in full orgasm whenever his own body releases into ejaculation.

⇒ Is Instant Orgasm an Improvement? ⇐

Instant coffee, fast foods, instant messaging—our society is one of instant gratification, of not having to wait and not wanting to waste time. We want everything at our fingertips and we want to do as little as possible to get the things we want. We want these things now, if not sooner. The dilemma is that brewed coffee tastes better than instant, and food cooked with care and to your specifications tastes better than fast food.

But not everything that is instant is necessarily a bad idea. Most people will agree that it is better to receive mail (especially checks) by airmail rather than by pony express. The speed with which we can communicate with almost everyone via the Internet is an improvement in most cases over having to wait for information; for example, information that traveled for months across the Atlantic Ocean by boat before the use of the telegraph.

What about instant orgasm? Is it an improvement? Or is it a cheap imitation of "normal" orgasm? Does it suffer in comparison to the old paradigm of a (usually) lengthy arousal period before reaching the point of no return? Is it better than the "wait, wait, tense up, tense up, and finally squirt" type of orgasm? Will it only last for ten seconds and then be done? Is an instant orgasm even possible?

Instant orgasm is about opening your mind to a new definition of orgasm. It is about being conscious and using that consciousness to feel. It is about putting your attention on your pleasure and focusing on the tactile sensations you are experiencing.

The trouble (if indeed it is "trouble") with instant orgasm, which we define as coming on or before the first stroke, is that it usually has to be learned. It has to be practiced. Fully comprehending and appreciating it takes time. For some people (almost always women), the mere idea of immediate orgasmic possibility triggers something in their mind that says, "I can do that." They find the idea itself so liberating that they are able to experience instant orgasm right away. This capability, however, is not what we have seen as the usual response. For most, it takes time and practice to attain the skill that a few "naturals" already possess. In our work training people to have extended massive orgasms (the topic of two of our earlier books), we are often asked how long it will take to be able to have one—or "How long before I can get off with the first stroke?" There is no exact way to predict. The answer is a combination of how willing the person is, how suggestible they are to new information, how sensual they are to begin with, whether they are used to using a vibrator (we discourage vibrators for serious sensual students as they tend to numb a person's nervous system rather than expanding sensation), how much priority they give to practicing, and whether they have a partner who is also interested in applying this new and provocative information.

I remember dancing with and even hugging some women, with both of us fully dressed, and feeling strong contractions in their bodies, most specifically around their genitals, just from the bodily contact. You have probably felt something similar, too, either directly as a woman or indirectly as a man. We define this response as an orgasm. So an instant orgasm is not as alien as you might think. I once had a sensual date with a woman who was responding orgasmically from hugging, yet when I got to her clitoris she actually turned off. This was probably because she was not trained to have an extended massive orgasm but could kind of sneak an orgasm in when she thought no one was looking. When she undressed and was supposed to be pleasured, she felt performance anxiety. We will discuss this phenomenon later.

The good news is that what you're practicing is receiving more pleasure. It is about reacquiring what we believe to have been an instinct we were born with but that has been conditioned out of us by our pleasure-denying, pain-oriented, and even "fuck-oriented" societies. This practicing of pleasure is a fun journey. All one has to do, as the saying goes, is to enjoy each step of the way. One does not have to get to where one is going right away, only to appreciate every little nuance of improvement. Take time to "smell the roses," as there will be lots of fine-smelling roses on this path. Sensuality is about feeling the pleasure, the good sensations that are happening in the moment. It is about *now*. Focusing one's attention on the pleasure one is feeling right now can yield explosive possibilities. We have so many nerve receptors in our pleasure areas. Deciding to use them for feeling what is occurring right now—and having that be the *only* goal—is a truly wonderful breakthrough. All your focus, all your energy, is being used for the purpose of exquisite sensation. If you slip into your head and start thinking about other matters or comparing past experiences to this one, just put your attention back on your pleasure. All you have to do is get back on the horse, as it were, and begin to feel again.

How Is Instant Orgasm Different from Extended Massive Orgasm?

In our books on extended massive orgasm (EMO) we included information on how to start orgasming on or before the first stroke. However, this information got somewhat lost in the perhaps more sensational details of orgasming for many minutes, or even for hours. We believe that the data about being instantly orgasmic is far too valuable to be missed, which is what compelled us to write this book. We want to make sure that this vitally important point is fully grasped by everyone. Until you understand and are able to experience orgasmic pleasure on or before the first stroke, you will not have a real EMO. We want you to be able to extend your orgasm so that it can be initiated at the beginning, the start, the commencement of the sensual experience. The ability to sustain an orgasm and the ability to feel orgasmic pleasure from the beginning are interrelated. To sustain the orgasm one has to be focused in the present moment, just as one has to be focused in the present moment to feel the first stroke.

The focus of this book is on the beginning, on that first stroke, on our ability as human beings to be present to a heck of a lot more pleasure than we have been led to believe we could experience. Subsequently, each stroke that comes after the first can be experienced with the same grand attention and appreciation, which is one of the key issues we will discuss. We will also delve deeper than ever before into how to keep the orgasm going. So even if you have read our earlier books on extended massive orgasm, there is additional information here to help you perfect your skills.

How, then, do we go about getting this instant orgasm? We read this book and say, "Wow, that would be great." We believe—we have faith—that it is possible. We practice, and we prioritize pleasure. We enjoy and savor every step.

⋙ Language and Orgasm ⋘

We would like for people to eventually consider changing the name of "instant orgasm" to simply "orgasm." Then the old kind of orgasm can be called just that—"the old kind of orgasm" (which we also affectionately refer to as a "crotch sneeze"). Why do this? We believe that you do not have to give up having the crotch-sneeze type of orgasm; we only suggest adding this new kind of pleasure to your repertoire. We call it a "crotch sneeze" more to get your attention than to demean it. It is comparable to a sneeze because it is over so quickly, but of course it can be very enjoyable. We also believe that when you practice this newer way of being orgasmic—that is, when you are instantly orgasmic and then experience wave after wave of orgasmic sensation—you will tend to prefer it, and you may or may not want to experience the old kind of orgasm any longer. However, the option will always be available. The phenomenon we're describing is analogous to the replacement of tube televisions with the high-definition, flat-screen variety. The picture is much more intense, and after a while the old TV may seem inferior—though it may be fun to see a black-and-white show once in a while. One day we will not have to use the adjective "HD" to describe TVs, just like we won't have to describe an orgasm as "extended massive" or "instant." It will simply be an "orgasm."

Language is likely the most important reason for our success as a species. Early on, it enabled us to hunt and gather food as a team, and to pass on knowledge that we gained through experiences. We do not have to go back to square one with each new generation; rather, through spoken and written language we can pass down many of our ideas and discoveries. However, when we have sex or create pleasure with someone, we are conditioned by our society to do it in the dark, using as little language as possible. Chapter 3 presents ways to talk with your partner that will enhance the experience.

⤜ New Thinking ⤛

Webster's defines "orgasm" as the climax of sexual tension, and this is the way most people understand the phenomenon. This definition means that you have to reach some threshold in order to have an orgasm. It also means that orgasm lasts for a very short time—a few seconds—and then ends. What if this concept itself is what is stopping us from experiencing a much fuller orgasm—waves of sensation that begin with the first stroke or even before, and last until the final stroke or even after?

What if our natural state is to be in orgasm all the time, and it is only when we move our attention to some other function or task that we do not experience these sensual feelings? Surviving in our world requires us to focus on different priorities at different times. We cannot sit around 24/7 getting off, being totally addicted to pleasure. We have other things to do. When a saber-toothed tiger was chasing our ancestors around the jungle it would not have been in their best interest to place all of their attention on orgasmic pleasures. When we are pounding a nail with a hammer it is best to focus on that nail—not on getting nailed. As the Bible says, there is a time and place for everything. The time and place for pleasure is whenever you want it and wherever it is in your best interest to have it.

Our puritanical heritage and religious conditioning, whether Christian or other, are largely responsible for keeping us from realizing that pleasure is an important part of life that is readily available and will not ruin our moral character. We are walking around with these glorious bodies and fantastically creative minds, and yet there is a culturally implanted V-chip that somehow prevents us from receiving the pleasure channel that is being sent to us at no charge from Mother Nature herself.

So the question becomes, how do we plug into that orgasmic channel? The answer, as you may have guessed, is by placing our attention on it. When our attention is on the pleasure of our genitals—on the wonderful sensations that titillate our largest organs, that is, our skin and our brains—when we can lower our defensive shields and raise our pleasure-sensing antennae, we will feel unadulterated pleasure. Likewise, when our attention is on the wrongness of pleasure or on the sinfulness of orgasmic bliss, we fail to feel the pleasure that is readily available to all of us in our natural state.

Our teacher, Dr. Vic Baranco, used to say that the whole world is in orgasm and all you have to do is plug into it. That sounds easy, yet it is an oversimplification, as there is no outlet like there is for plugging in your toaster. We have to intentionally create our connection with the cosmic orgasm by placing our focus on our pleasure centers and on not becoming distracted by judging ourselves based on how we compare or how we think we should feel. We cannot be pissed off at our partners and still have enough space in our consciousness for great fun. We are limited beings in that we can only confront and be aware of a small part of our universe at one time. It is either pleasure or something else, and our society gives us plenty of reasons why it is best to focus on something else.

So one of the first steps on this blissful journey is to realize that we have been brainwashed not to feel as much as we can—that we have been taught to avoid experiencing orgasmic sensations from birth onward. It is also important to realize that there is hope that we can experience this ecstasy, which Vera and I believe is every human's birthright. Our bodies can and do work wonderfully, given just a little mental adjustment and a little practice to restore what has lain dormant due to negative cultural conditioning from parents, peers, clergy, teachers, and others.

When a person realizes that they can feel ecstasy whenever they feel like it—that to achieve an orgasm they do not need to be in some ideal setting, or to wait for the perfect time, or to be inebriated—they are freed and their minds are opened.

This blissful journey is not a difficult one; it is a continually fascinating and creative passage with no destination, as such. It is ongoing, and it becomes part of who we are. This does not mean that we cannot or will not attempt other endeavors or that we will become so addicted to pleasure that we forget the rest of our lives. No—in fact, tuning in to pleasure will expand one's creativity in all aspects of being. It is a form of enlightenment, and as the Zen Buddhists say, "Before enlightenment, chop wood and carry water; after enlightenment, chop wood and carry water." Those daily tasks will just become that much more enjoyable.

The ability to be instantly orgasmic, especially for women, actually frees up a person's time and thoughts. One no longer has to be concerned about their sexual aptitude, as they have already passed the test. This does not mean that one's capacity for pleasure will not grow or get better, but it does signify that the tiger is no longer being swung by its tail. Now the tail is being moved when and if the tiger so desires. This is very freeing to women who have been kept in the dark for so long about their sexual aptitude and fulfillment. Once a woman knows she can get off whenever and for however long she desires, there is no further need for her to be concerned about her orgasmic ability. She can focus her energy and creativity on other endeavors without entertaining this nagging doubt. And when a man learns how to produce this pleasure for a woman, he is also freed. He becomes more confident and self-assured and can concentrate on other things, again without any doubt about his sexual skills nagging at him and blurring his focus.

⇒ Women and Men Differ in Response ⇐

We teach a class called the DEMO, which stands for Demonstration of an Extended Massive Orgasm. In it we demonstrate a manually induced, hour-long orgasm on a woman. This live presentation is given in front of a mixed audience of men and women. Everyone can see the woman's intense orgasm, and many students are even allowed to come to the front of the room so they can touch her leg or stomach. Many of the women in the class can feel orgasmic sensations in their own genitals while they view the demonstration. They report getting wet and having contractions (i.e., being orgasmic) without any genital contact. Although the men can observe the sensations that are occurring in the woman demonstrator, their bodies do not respond in the same manner as those of the female students.

As mentioned, we believe that women are the source of turn-on, and that a heterosexual man can and will respond to a woman who is using her turn-on to stimulate him via her thoughts, pheromones, or whatever (the actual means have not yet been scientifically determined). The men in our classes who are in a room of turned-on women are not yet turned on themselves as there is no female energy directed specifically at them. The women in the room turn themselves on; this is one of the innate functions they possess that men lack. On occasion, a woman, sometimes one of the teachers but usually one of the students, will have a sexual thought or fantasy about a man or men in general, and many of the men (and also most of the women) will feel this as pleasure in their genitals, usually in the form of erectile activity in their penises. Women are therefore the source of pleasure for themselves and for men, and sometimes for other women.

Although women seem to have a greater capacity for self-created pleasure and for influencing men to think about pleasure, this in no way means that men must wait for the influence of some feminine charm before they can experience pleasure. A man can have a wet dream without any penile stimulation. He can fantasize, through either thoughts or pictures. He can touch himself and feel pleasure. The amount of pleasure he can experience on the first stroke depends on how much attention he's placing on what he is feeling, and also upon what kind of expectations and views he entertains about orgasm. Is he touching himself in a relaxed way, or is he just doing it to relieve himself of sexual tension? When a woman turns her dial up and lasers it toward a man, he can feel very intense pleasure; we can call this an instant orgasm. It is somewhat out of his control, yet his ability to focus on his pleasure can amplify her signals or dampen them if he remains unconscious of them.

So there seem to be some differences as well as some similarities between how men and women experience sensual pleasure, specifically instant orgasm.

⋙ The Old Kind of Orgasm ⋘

When most people think of orgasm they think of the graph created by Masters and Johnson showing four distinct parts of the sensual experience: excitement, plateau (arousal), orgasm, and resolution. These occur in the old paradigm wherein a person remains tensed up while being stimulated because they are waiting for the end goal of orgasm. But we ask, what really separates excitement and arousal from orgasm? This is key to the concept of instant orgasm.

As we see it, people's sexual response is completely subject to what they believe about it—that is, how they view the experience based on what they have been taught and what they have seen others do. Most of what people, both men and women, have seen is actually the male orgasm. He tenses up, tenses up, tenses up, and then squirts, squirts, squirts, and then he can go no farther. How many women have ever seen another woman have an orgasm? Women base their own idea of what they think their orgasms should be like on the orgasms had by the males they have been in bed with or have seen in movies or porn films.

This has been a successful sexual response for men as it feels good, especially the ejaculatory phase. The problem is that most women do not have this same ejaculatory phase. They do, however, have a greater capacity for feeling sensation then men do, as the clitoris has a higher concentration of nerve endings than does any portion of the male anatomy. The sole function of the clitoris is to experience pleasure. Many modern women are aware that their clitorises are where the action is. They either masturbate there or, when engaged in partnered sex, require their lovers to stimulate it. This is definitely a step in the right direction, but we have noticed that most women are still trying to experience orgasm in the same way men do. They tense their bodies and hope to eventually come or even ejaculate.

We consistently get e-mails from women and some men (about their partners) who are concerned about not being orgasmic while having intercourse. We would have thought that the word had gotten around by now informing women about how their bodies work and about the low percentages of women who actually have coital orgasms. We guess Dr. Freud had a bigger influence than we'd hoped in this arena. He stated that there were two types of orgasm, vaginal and clitoral, and that the vaginal kind was "superior" to the clitoral kind. This apparent misconception still influences many people's thinking on the matter. Simply put, there is no such thing as a vaginal orgasm as there are no proprioceptive nerve endings in the vaginal wall surface. Of course, through our teachings and those of others, a woman can learn to feel more and include stimulation of her clitoris in the coital act, thereby leading to an orgasm. It is not a vaginal orgasm. It is clitorally based, as are all female orgasms.

Many women feel inferior because they do not have vaginal orgasms, yet their clitoral orgasms really are the standard itself and these women just don't know it. The Hollywood film industry—which depicts coitus as a fantastic sexual romp with the man on top, and then the woman, and then the man again—is promoting a fiction that has prejudiced women and men into thinking that they should be able to duplicate this wonderful experience in their own bedrooms. Yet they fail to find the gratification that was promised.

We promise you something better, something real, and something that at first you will find mind-blowing: an orgasm that starts the explosion with the first touch. As we've stated, we think that eventually an EMO will be considered the norm and that the notion of a woman imitating a man by going for the tensed-up, seconds-long orgasmic release will be in the minority. Then maybe men will be able to imitate the way women orgasm, thereby increasing their pleasure, too. This orgasmic eruption does not require a great deal of kindling and, like a nuclear reactor, can keep producing energy for an extended period of time.

⮞ First Step ⮜

The first step in having an instant orgasm is realizing that it is possible. If you've never heard of something or considered it a possibility, that thing has no place in your mind. It just doesn't exist. Your mind is filled with symbols and triggers to other symbols encompassing everything you have learned or imagined, and if you have never heard of instantaneous orgasmic response then to you it doesn't exist. In order to even entertain a new idea, one has to first be made aware of it. It's kind of like when people used to think the world was flat. If you had told them that it was round they would have thought you were crazy and probably a troublemaker. Or it's like when Galileo tried to convince people that Copernicus was correct in thinking the earth revolved around the sun instead of vice versa. Despite recanting this belief in the face of the Spanish Inquisition he was placed under house arrest for years and narrowly missed being executed for his radical ideas.

Even better than reading or hearing about the possibility of an immediate orgasmic response is getting to see one for yourself. As mentioned, we give live demonstrations showing that a person can reach an orgasmic state very quickly. We also do hands-on work (pardon the pun) with individual students and sometimes with couples, usually in our apartment. Both Vera and I are always present for these person-to-person sessions. There are quite a few people now living on our planet who can orgasm deliberately from the first stroke and who even teach this technique, so the idea is slowly spreading (just like any useful meme or information virus, as Richard Dawkins would call it). The tipping point has not yet been reached, so the idea of instant orgasm remains unknown to most. Hopefully this book will help spread the word.

When people see it with their own eyes, they are usually convinced that coming on the first stroke is a real phenomenon. Some still may think that it is some kind of trick or fakery, but at least they have opened their minds to the possibility of the experience, and that is a step in the right direction. They have created a symbol for the occurrence in their minds, so at least they can think about it.

We recently met some women who said that IO and EMO are impossible for them, yet they had never witnessed either one! That kind of negative prejudice can keep people from experiencing something fantastic. The positive news is that at least now they have been exposed to the concepts. Although they haven't embraced the possibility for themselves, by having heard of the phenomena they are ahead of where they were.

➢ Check It Out for Yourself ➣

Once people see that instant orgasm is not only possible but fairly easy to achieve, many will try it. As we've said, it takes some practice to change old habits—to switch from tensing up and thus not feeling much during a sensual encounter to relaxing and feeling as much as one can. Therefore, the second step in creating an IO is to practice doing it. You can practice by yourself or with a partner. Perhaps it is best to try both ways. The next chapter describes several ways to practice by yourself, and later chapters detail techniques for practicing with a partner.

When you receive pleasure from either your own hand or that of a partner, it is important to approve of all the sensations you feel. That is, don't judge any feeling, or yourself, as wrong or inadequate; just be aware of the sensation without evaluating it in any way. Know that the intensity of the sensation will be less powerful on the first stroke than it will as you continue the stimulation. The intensity gets stronger as you go along, and the best and fastest way to get there is by approving of what you are experiencing right now, not by tensing or ignoring the present moment for the hope of coming in the future. Instead of going to the symphony to listen to the last ten seconds of music, you go to listen to the entire performance. You hear and feel each note and combination of instruments, and you especially pay attention to the opening sounds, which enrich your mind after stimulating your ears.

The genitals of both men and women contain a lot of nerve endings. They can feel the air; they can even feel a hand that is held just above them without touching the skin. They can feel heat and cold. They are highly sensitive, and with practice and attention they become even more receptive and responsive. Combined with a willing mind, they can eagerly anticipate and easily feel.

Every sensual experience is different. The more positive a person's past experiences, the easier he or she will find it to be pleasured the next time. It isn't necessary to try to repeat the same experience each time out; in fact, doing so can produce problems, like comparing the present moment to a memory, which causes one's awareness to be focused on judging instead of feeling the stroke at hand.

We have observed that the most difficult part of having an instant orgasm is the first step: embracing the concept itself. People are so used to waiting for climax that even when they feel pleasurable sensations on the first stroke, they do not think they are in orgasm. They assume orgasm has to be something equivalent to male ejaculation. We have written about this natural ability in our other books, yet some who have read them did not get the concept. They still thought they had to wait to feel orgasmic pleasure. Once they do get it, especially our women students, they take off. They love it that there is no place they have to get to, that it is all about what is going on right now. It is so liberating to tap into a potential that before had lain dormant. There it is on the first stroke, or even before. You don't have to get anywhere—just feel it right now, right there on the clitoris. Most of our students feel it when we merely say the words, "Feel your clitoris." To watch a woman remember her power, to see her turn on and light up just for the fun of doing so, is a thrilling experience.

Another Difference Between Women and Men

We have had female students read their erotic journals to us. Vera, who is easy to turn on, would often feel the words in her genitals. We have found that women in general are more influenced by words, whether spoken or written, than men are. This is why many women like romance novels and most men just don't get them. Many men are visually stimulated, so viewing an erotic pose could perhaps do the same for them. When our students read their journals aloud I would report that the turn-on did not reach me. They would reread the same sentences with more feeling in their genitals, and *then* I could pick up the sensation in my loins. This was a huge "aha" moment for the women in the group, for now they realized that all they had to do was feel the pleasure themselves and the man would also be able to feel it. Vera, or any other woman who is aware of her innate ability, could turn herself on with the erotic words. It didn't even matter if the student wasn't feeling it. This shows how important it is for men to learn how to speak and write in ways that will be appreciated by women, and for women to realize that the way they feel can have a powerful effect on men (whether or not words are involved).

So a woman can instantly turn herself on whenever she decides to. Men cannot do so just by willing it. A man can use his mind and fantasize about something that turns him on, or he can use his visual receptors and look at pictures or videos that he finds stimulating. Some men can become confused about whether they are getting turned on by fantasizing or by the woman they are with. It is usually by the woman, but not always, and just because she is turning him on does not give him any "rights" to use his erection on her unless she gives him more direct information. He can ask her questions if the situation warrants it, or he can just enjoy the pleasure of being turned on by her without mentioning it to her. Each situation is unique, and men have to learn which approach is most appropriate in different kinds of circumstances. The more a man has sex, including self-pleasuring, the less of a sense of scarcity he will attach to sex, and this will free him up to act in everyone's best interest.

~

The next chapter explores a number of different avenues for self-pleasuring. It describes how to create an IO in your own body and how to expand on those sensations, especially in women, and it gives men ways to enhance the amount of pleasure they can feel, too.

CHAPTER 2

Self-Pleasure

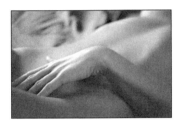

*T*his chapter begins by exploring humans' ability to deliberately focus attention on pleasurable tactile sensations—an ability we have with each of our five senses. It also touches on our capacity for conceptual (imaginative) thought. We are presenting you with the tools for having instant orgasms. We outline exercises to enhance this ability; for some, doing the exercises will trigger instant orgasms. The second part of the chapter describes exercises for increasing your body's ability to feel extended pleasure with the first stroke and beyond, with special emphasis on building connections between your genitals and the rest of your body.

⮞ Receptivity ⮜

As we've discussed, a person who wishes to experience an instant orgasm must first be receptive to the idea. In the last chapter we considered how our minds can become open to this concept. Now we will focus on how our minds influence our bodies. You must get your body into the receptive mode. You have to place your attention on your body's tactile sensations, and you have to refocus your attention on these sensations whenever you have extraneous thoughts. This means placing your attention on your genitals; this is how you create the desire and the sensation. Our nervous system is constantly inundated with all kinds of sensual overload, and our brains usually unconsciously decide which sensations to allow us to notice and which ones to keep us from noticing.

Our consciousness is only able to perceive a small amount of the sensation that is bombarding us; the rest is lost. In addition, our minds are cluttered with extraneous thoughts and past losses. I know for myself that when something negative occurs in my personal universe I tend to dwell on it, foregoing any positive movement forward. We have to make a concerted effort to put our attention on something pleasurable.

We are also difference-sensing beings; that is, our attention is drawn to a change in stimulation. If there is a change in what you smell—for example, a woman walks into your presence wearing fresh perfume—you will notice it, but only for a while. You will notice a loud noise, but if it continues at a steady frequency, at some point you will no longer be as keenly aware of it.

We humans have the ability to override this internal censor and focus our attention on any specific sense. Most of the time, even though our sense of touch is being stimulated, we do not notice it, as our unconscious censor is keeping us focused on some other sense or on some negative thought. Did you feel your buttocks on the chair until you read this sentence? We thought not.

By deliberately training ourselves to feel the potential pleasure in our genitals we can feel much more than we think is possible—and this ability expands with use. We can learn to silence most of our other senses and to concentrate on specific pleasures of the genitals. However, we are generally so used to being on the lookout for negative stimuli, such as pain or discomfort, that it may take some time to grasp the idea of receiving pleasurable stimuli anytime we desire.

⤳ Focusing Your Attention ⤲

The ability to feel pleasure whenever you so desire and wherever you are may very well be innate to all of us; however, by the time we are adults it is usually forgotten. When we are newborns our skin loves to be touched. Our baby nervous system "connects" much of our skin so that being touched feels good all over our body. As we grow up we learn to differentiate one area of our body from another, and the old nerve connections fall out of use. Without use, the nerves fail to send signals as often or as well as they once did, and these pathways atrophy. From a functional viewpoint, this is actually a positive change that helps us to determine what area of our body is being touched and to respond correctly. One does not want to pull one's foot away from the hot stove if one's hand is burning. The downside is that we feel less overall; we are not pleasured all over, but rather only in restricted areas—one area at a time if we are lucky.

Here's a major concept behind instant orgasm: You can actually have both the functional (compartmentalized) and the pleasurable (connected) nervous system available to you at all times if you are willing to practice certain skills.

There are a number of exercises that can bring back the ability to feel sensation all over the body from the experience of a single touch. These involve developing the ability to properly focus your attention. Some of the exercises may seem simple, yet practicing them repeatedly is usually required to bring results for most people. There is no strict timetable that fits everybody, but if you continue these exercises we can say that you will become more proficient at feeling more pleasure in less time. Many of our women students are happily surprised at how much they can actually feel when given the permission to do so.

Here's a simple exercise to get you started. At any time of the day when you think it is safe to do so, place your attention on your genitals for a few seconds with the intention of feeling as much pleasure as you can. You can use different associations to remind you to practice—for example, when you are stopped at a red light. (You may even start to look forward to red lights instead of feeling negative about them.) Or perhaps you can practice just before you open a door. These practice episodes take only a few seconds of your time. The best time to do them is when you are not focusing on any other activity; therefore, it is better to do them at a red light instead of when you are driving. This way you can put all of your attention on any sensation you feel. Do not expect to feel a great amount of sensation at first. Approve of any sensation you feel, even if it is just a little heat or a minute amount of feeling or tingling. Other examples of good times to practice include while watching a commercial on TV (or perhaps given the inane nature of many of today's TV shows it may be a good time to put your attention on your body while the show itself is being aired) or when you see someone attractive as you are walking down the street. (For our women readers, know that the latter example could be risky, as people may respond to a woman who is feeling turned on. This may be better advice for a man than for a woman.)

Reading is another time when people are usually alone, and it can be a splendid occasion to practice feeling immediate sensation. Try doing it at the end of a page or at the end of a chapter. Whenever you come to the end of some logical division in a book, feel free to focus on your genitals for a few seconds. As a matter of fact, right now would be a perfect time to start this practice. Put the book down for a few seconds, close your eyes (if you like), and place your attention on feeling as much pleasurable sensation in your pussy or penis as possible.

We are glad that you have begun your training in becoming instantly orgasmic. Regardless of how much or how little you felt just now, you are on the path. Be creative about when and where you do this noticing. We have given you a number of ideas; you are free to choose among them and, of course, to come up with your own.

➤ Ways of Touching Yourself ➤

This section suggests several ways to experiment with touching yourself. For both men and women, instant orgasm is about noticing and maximizing the initial burst of sensation that occurs when you first focus your attention on your genitals. So for the sake of these activities, we want you to feel the sensations for a second or so and then stop. You can repeat each exercise as often as you care to. The goal is to feel increased sensation from the get-go; the more often you do this, the better you will become at feeling from the first stroke. So start and stop, start and stop, and so on.

In the Tub or Shower

A good time to play with your sensations could be in a Jacuzzi or bathtub as you let the water flow over your genitals. The shower is another great place to experience some intentional instant pleasuring. You are naked, no one is around, and it is easy to focus on different parts of your body. You can start by feeling the air on your pleasure spots. Then you can feel the water from the showerhead against your genitals. Proceed in an on-and-off manner, for not too long—and see if you can become pleasured with just a little attention. You can touch yourself with the bar of soap or with your hand, just touching, not necessarily stroking. Feel the pleasure, and approve of what you feel. We predict that you will at least feel the beginnings of tingling sensations.

With a Water Hose

The water hose is a great accessory for women who are seriously interested in exploring their sensuality. The hose can be a simple rubber tube attached to the bathtub faucet. Some hoses come with a showerhead; you can simply cut off the spray portion and leave the small-bored water hose. Some tubs won't fit a simple accessory; if that's the case then you'll have to go to the hardware store and get a special attachment. You can tell the salesperson that you want an attachment to hose off your pet in the tub. This small investment can go a long way.

Once you have obtained your hose, fill your tub with a few inches of warm water and play with the water flowing from the hose. For women, this is a great replacement for a vibrator, which can numb the nerves. Lying back, aim the hose at your vulva and clitoral area. Play with the pressure by either changing the amount of water released from the faucet or pinching the hose. This may take some getting used to, so please give this exercise more than one try. We know of many women who dearly love their baths.

Another water possibility is the bidet. Most European homes have one, but few American homes do. Some luxury hotels have them. The water temperature and pressure can be adjusted, and if you get into the right position you can aim the water flow directly at your most sensual areas.

Whether you're using a hose or a bidet, play with your initial feelings by aiming the water directly at the different areas of your genitals for only a short time. Check out your labia, your perineum, your anus, and of course your clitoris, with the hood both in place and retracted. See which areas spark the most sensation. Later you can graduate to keeping the water aimed at your genitals for longer amounts of time, but right now we are especially interested in getting you to feel more sensation from the very first, and slightest, moment of contact.

Using Fantasy

It is okay to fantasize if it heightens what you feel. This may work better for men, as most women have longer, more involved fantasies that take time to develop, and again the goal is to feel the sensation now and to feel it quickly. Furthermore, whereas women can turn on at will, men require a woman to become turned on, or they use some other force, such as a touch or a fantasy, if no woman is interested or available. A few paragraphs above we mentioned how men can feel pleasurable sensations in their genitals when they pass a pretty woman. Some men can also direct attention on their crotch when they see an attractive woman on TV. Many men will already have been doing this, as men are very visual and can fantasize easily. The point here is to do it deliberately, do it only for a few seconds, and then stop and repeat, if desired. We want you to gain more control over these sensations and to learn how to create them whenever you want to. Do not, of course, interact with a woman on the street when you are in this mode, as the goal is for you to feel, not to find a relationship. If finding a relationship is your goal then your attention must be placed elsewhere.

Women, if you want to interact with some stranger on the street—which most women do not want to do—then it may be okay to place your attention on your pussy. However, this could get you into trouble, so, again, we do not recommend it.

With Your Hand (and Other Objects)

Another way to put attention on your genitals is to touch yourself. This is especially useful for men, who tend to require more direct stimulation. Touch yourself either through your clothes, or while naked, or with an additional barrier such as a pillow on top of your genital area. You can play with different amounts of hand pressure, or just allow yourself to feel the pressure of the pillow. You could also put the pillow between your legs and squeeze it. You may have heard of girls who get pleasure from riding a horse. Vera, who grew up in Europe, says that when she was around twelve years old she would ride the trains and would feel pleasure in her genitals from the vibration of the seat. Our genitals are stocked with nerve endings, and a little bit of sensation can go a long way.

I remember a history teacher who would put his leg over the back of a chair and rub his genitals back and forth as he talked. This may not be such a great idea these days, with all the fears about child molesters and indecent exposure; however, he was certainly enjoying himself, perhaps out of habit, and he may not even have known he was doing it. Nowadays he would probably be better off doing it in the privacy of his own home.

In the Bedroom

The privacy granted by your own bedroom makes it one of the best settings for touching yourself. You can use fantasy or not, depending on how you respond to it. You can use pornography, if that floats your boat, or just use mental images and ideas. Again, the goal is not to sustain the pleasure for any length of time but to feel as much as you can from the first placement of attention on your genitals. Men do not have to be erect to feel pleasure, and, in fact, the more mental pressure they put on themselves in this regard the more difficult it becomes to get hard. Women do not have to be steaming hot either; they just need to be in the feeling mode and to approve of all sensations. Again, you can do this through your clothes or naked, or start with your clothes on and then peel off your pants or skirt. Then touch yourself through your underwear, and eventually take those off, too. You do not need any lubricant for this exercise, as you are not stroking, just touching.

A useful idea, prior to touching yourself, is to first focus all your energy and attention on the area to be touched. Make that area ready, anticipating, and eager for any touch. Be experimental. Check out as many different types of touch as you can think of—from light to firm pressure, using only a fingertip, then your whole finger, then your whole hand. Touch a small area and then a larger area. Touch for a split second or longer, keeping the pressure on any pleasurable area of your genitals for as long as you like—that is, for as long as it keeps feeling wonderful.

For Guys

If you are a man, try putting your hand around your penis and giving yourself gentle squeezes, releasing and squeezing again. Again, this can be done directly on the skin or through your clothes. By doing it through your clothes you place less stress on yourself to take the pleasure to a certain place; you are just doing it for the fun of the moment. As we stated previously, an erection isn't necessary; however, if one does occur that's fine too. I've touched myself through my clothes without any expectations—just some repeated, gentle, one-second squeezes and releases. It feels so good that I often become erect and sometimes even leak a significant amount of semen. Although this is not an ejaculation, it might be even better than one. You can continue to squeeze or do other pleasurable things to your penis because you are not overly sensitized as you would be if you had fully ejaculated, in which case you would not want to continue being touched there. By stimulating yourself without ejaculating, if you were to have some fun in bed with another person later on, you would be easily aroused and would not have any discomfort. As men get older they generally do not ejaculate as often as men in their teens or twenties. One ejaculation a day is enough for most, and even that might be pushing it for some men. When they have more ejaculations than their bodies can appreciate, men can actually feel pain or become desensitized. Merely touching for the pleasure of it, not stroking to reach ejaculation, is another way to appreciate sensuality. At some point in your training you may want to check out squeezing, with the addition of some lubricant.

As we have repeatedly stated, an erect penis is not necessary for experiencing a great deal of pleasure, except during intercourse. Nor is ejaculation

necessary for orgasm (as we define it). Ejaculation is only the end of the orgasm, not the whole orgasm. Ejaculation is only crucial for fertilizing an egg,
which is not essential to orgasm and pleasure. In fact, it can be detrimental to
extended pleasure. Of course, a really splendid ejaculation via a fully erect penis, with insertion or without, can feel wonderful and can be a fitting end to
the sexual experience. It just is not necessary.

I have to admit that throughout my life I have been an ejaculator; that is,
I've almost always finished a sexual act, whether with my partner or with myself, by ejaculating. Since I've been writing this book I've been practicing not
finishing every masturbation session with an ejaculation. This has enabled
me to masturbate more often for short periods, and when I have sex with Vera
I actually feel more than ever before. In one sense I'm not really masturbating, as I am not doing any stroking, just using the touches we have described.
I guess some people would call it fore-masturbation. There is a time and place
for all kinds of sexual and sensual experiences, and hopefully we are adding
to what you are already doing by giving you some new and different options.
If you are doing these things already, we are certainly putting our stamp of approval on them.

For Gals

As we've stated, women can feel a lot of pleasure and even be orgasmic simply
by focusing their attention on their genitals. Of course, this does not preclude
touching themselves, whether with their own hand, water, or some other object. Here we present you with a few ideas for practicing various touches.
Create a space where you will not be disturbed so you can play with yourself
without anyone bothering you. Bear in mind that it is still important to focus
your attention on your pleasure areas when you are touching yourself.

A woman's clitoris has more nerve endings than any other place on her
body and therefore has the potential for generating the most sensation. In
addition, there are other areas nearby that have a lot of nerve endings, too;
these include the perineum, the inner vulval lips, the introitus, and the anus
(see Figure 1). Really, a woman's entire genital region is quite sensitive, and a
woman can play with any one of these areas.

Figure 1.
Female genitals

mons ——————————

clitoral hood ——————————
clitoris ——————————

introitus ——————————
inner labia ——————————

outer labia ——————————
perineum ——————————
anus ——————————

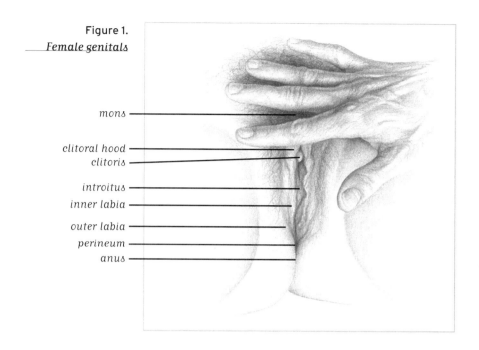

Through your clothing, through your panties, or directly on your naked body, you can touch whatever area you feel like touching. Again, the goal is to feel as much as you can for a short time and then to remove your hand. The more you can approve of any positive sensations you feel, the better your ability to increase the amount of sensation. So touch, feel, remove, and enjoy. Repeat this sequence for as long as it is fun to do so. You can touch the same spot over and over or move to a new spot whenever you like. If touching a specific spot feels great, it is okay to keep your hand there for as long as the wonderful sensation lasts.

As we've said, a woman can direct pleasure to her genitals without having to fantasize or be touched. You can combine this pleasurable, targeted attention with touches to make the sensations even more exquisite. Turn on an area or spot by placing your attention on it, feel the sensations, and then touch it to add even more feeling. Approve of all sensation you experience. Then remove your hand and start over again, if you would like to do so.

Another activity is to squeeze your clitoris through the hood, using two fingers (see Figure 11 on page 94), to squeeze and release. The clitoris can actually receive a great deal of pressure and still feel fantastic. Do not squeeze with too much pressure at first; gradually increase the pressure each time you squeeze. You do not have to remove your fingers after each squeeze; just back off and then repeat with added pressure. Learn which amount of pressure you most prefer. Notice if you have any engorgement in the area.

Some women feel that their clitoris is too sensitive to be touched at all. Some of these women can accept having the clitoris touched through the hood, while others may be afraid to do even that. In our research we have not met any women who, after some training, continued to reject having their clitoris touched directly or through the hood. Reaching this point can take time, so if you feel very sensitive, go slowly and cautiously and you will learn to accept more and more sensation there. This is your time to experiment. Go as fast or as slow as you wish. Use as much pressure as feels good to you. As you treat yourself respectfully with regard to your feelings, your attitude about your sensitivity will begin to change.

Try pulling and stretching your genitals in any direction and using any amount of pressure that feels good. You can spread apart your inner labia (labia minora) using two hands (see Figure 2), or you can put pressure on your mons pubis, above the clitoris, pulling upward and pushing into the body using varying amounts of pressure (see Figure 3). You can pull your hood back and expose your clitoris with one hand or both hands, using one or more fingers (see Figure 4). Again, this is your playtime, so experiment with every method of exposing the clitoris that you can think of. Feel the air flowing over your clitoris as you reveal it from its covering.

Figure 2.
Spreading apart the
inner labia

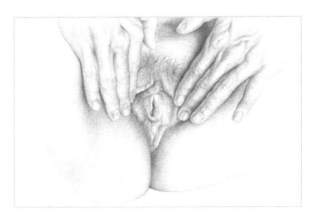

Figure 3.
*Applying pressure
to the mons area*

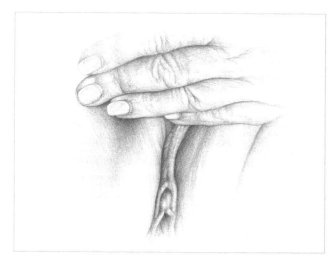

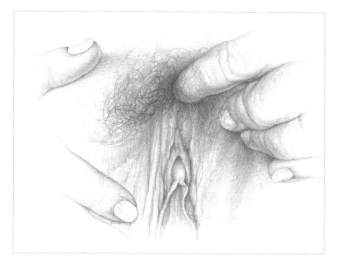

Figure 4.
*Exposing the
clitoris*

Try exposing your clitoris and then, with your other hand, touch the clitoral head for just a brief moment. If you are able to do so, check out how it feels to touch different areas of your clitoris. We like to divide the head of the clitoris into quadrants: the upper and lower left and the upper and lower right. There is also an upper middle and a lower middle, as well as a bottom area. You can touch each of these using different amounts of pressure and from different angles. Everyone's clitoris is different. Some women have larger ones that are easier to divide into areas, and some women have very small ones that are impossible to divide up, except for maybe left and right sides. What is important here is to see how *your* clitoris likes to be touched and, if possible, to discover what part of your clitoris feels best when touched and what kinds of pressure you prefer. There is no wrong or right way to touch yourself. Just experiment with brief touches—no stroking yet.

Notice the wetness of your inner lips and introitus with the tip of your finger, or even with your full finger placed parallel to the labia. Touch with any part of your finger, the underside or the edge. You can use your knuckles, or the base of your palm, or any part of your hand, front or back or side. Check out the top of your labia where they almost touch the clitoris. To test the sensation in smaller areas, like a specific spot on your labia, it is best to use your fingertip. Compare the sensation between the lower and middle portion of your inner labia. Determine which areas are most sensitive and which feel the most pleasure when touched.

For Both Men and Women

A type of touch that both men and women can enjoy is to briefly stroke the inner thighs. Place a hand palm-down on each thigh. Or, rather than using the palm, you can use the back of the hand. The action is more of a stroke than just a touch or a squeeze, but no lubrication is necessary as this is not erectile tissue. Starting from the genital area, quickly and fairly lightly stroke downward toward the knee. You can also start near the knee and stroke upward toward the genitals. The goal, again, is to feel as much as possible in a short time. After stroking once or twice, take a break and appreciate any sensations. Repeat the stroking action if it feels good to you.

You can also place your fingers on your thighs, pads down, and press without stroking. It can be fun to get close to your genitals without touching them and press inward on the inner thigh, alternating between left and right. This can set up a kind of link between the thighs, causing wonderful sensations to pass through the genitals. Use two, three, or four fingertips on each thigh, and press for just a second. Then release and do the same on your other thigh. You can try touching different spots on your inner thighs, moving your hands closer and then farther away from your genitals in a kind of teasing manner. You can vary the pressure to determine what feels best. You can alternate between pressing and lightly stroking. We want you to learn how to feel plea-sure from many kinds of tactile stimulation, and we want you to increase your ability to feel from the very first moment of contact. The touching, coupled with your focused attention, will create greater pleasurable sensations, espe-cially the more you practice these exercises.

Many other body parts enjoy being touched by you or by someone else. It can be very pleasurable to briefly touch your stomach or neck. I love pressing down on my lower abdomen with quite a bit of pressure and then releasing the pressure and repeating the action following a regular rhythm. Doing this feels good before I start masturbating and feels even better after I have been masturbating for some time (see Figure 5). Again, experiment with different amounts of pressure.

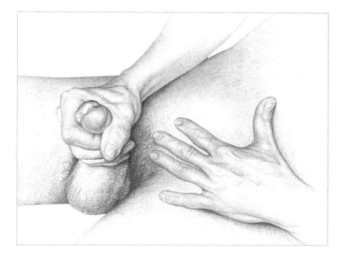

Figure 5.
Pressing on
abdomen while
stroking penis

The anal area is endowed with many nerve endings, containing the second highest concentration of nerve endings after the penis or clitoris. Touching the anal area can feel wonderfully sensational. With or without lubricant, you can play around with the whole area using varying amounts of pressure, dif-ferent types of squeezes, and one or more fingers. Try doing this through your clothing or underwear or even naked. Start by touching yourself at a fair dis-tance from your anus, and gradually move your touches closer. Some people may be squeamish about the anus, so respect your own personal boundaries. Penetration is not necessary here. These exercises are meant to be enjoyed.

Sometimes it is okay to push your envelope further than you think you would like, and other times you know when you are going too far.

⋙ More Exercises ⋘

In our EMO books we included an exercise called "Connections." During this exercise a person strokes his or her penis or clitoris (which we call the primary area) at the same time as they are stroking another body part (the secondary area). Many students don't go as far as they might with this practice. The results are subtle and usually take some time to manifest. People who don't see any big, instant changes often stop practicing before giving the exercise a chance and therefore fail to gain the full benefit.

This exercise is extremely important if a person wants to feel more sensation at any time they choose. If you want to become orgasmic on the first stroke, or simply by focusing your attention on your pleasure areas, it will be very helpful to create connections between a number of different body parts. The more connections you've developed and the deeper they are, the more sensation you can feel. Your body will become highly sensitive; you will notice subtle tingles and stirrings. Overall, you will become more aware of your tactile nervous system in a pleasurable way.

In addition to the connections exercise, we have gone into great detail in our previous books describing a series of preliminary exercises, including setting up a private space, taking a visual inventory of your body, taking a tactile inventory of your body, and using masturbation for pleasurable effect. All of these are very important, so they bear repeating here for readers who haven't been exposed to our earlier books. This section and the next one outline these exercises.

Before beginning these exercises, go to the drugstore and check out a few different types of lubricant. We usually use Albolene, an unscented makeup remover that has a thinner consistency than Vaseline. As both Albolene and Vaseline are petroleum-based products, they are not compatible with condoms. We also like K-Y Jelly and Astroglide, which are water-soluble. Water-based lubes tend to get sticky after they've been on the body for a while. If you use a water-based lube, have a cup of warm water nearby to dip your fingers into when the lubricant starts getting tacky.

Setting Up Your Space

The object here is to create a space where you can do your exercises in private, with no interruptions. The bedroom is probably the first choice, though we have had students who have used the bathroom or other places. Fix up your space so that it is visually appealing. Add pretty items, like flowers or candles, and include a tasty treat and something to drink. Also add an item that is pleasant to touch (such as a silk scarf), music you enjoy, and an appealing fragrance (incense, scented candles, essential oils, a rose). Finally, bring in any fantasy, romance novel, or pornography that you desire. You will require a full-length mirror and a hand mirror as well as some lubricant and towels.

You do not have to spend much time creating your space; thirty minutes should be more than enough. We have known people who have spent all day fixing up their space and then were too tired to do anything else.

This exercise is in some ways the most important of all because it sets the tone for the others, so do not skip it. And again, make sure that you will not be disturbed.

Visual Inventory

We believe it is vital for a person to enjoy who they are physically; we want you to fall in love with yourself and your body. The best present you can give your partner is a turned-on body, and if you do not like your body you will not get turned on easily. This exercise is extremely useful in learning to appreciate and love yourself and the way you look. The object is to look at yourself in the mirror and notice what you like about your body. Usually we look into a mirror to see what is wrong; for instance, to determine whether our hair is out of place or if we have a zit on our chin. For the purpose of this exercise, look into the mirror to determine what you like about your body. Start by noticing anything that strikes you in a positive way. It can be any part of your body as long as you like or love it. The more parts of your body you can approve of, the easier it will be to approve of more. Learn to love yourself the way you are; don't focus on how you think you should look or compare yourself to some unreal supermodel. Use the full-length mirror and the hand mirror to see yourself from many different angles. Do this exercise for as long as you enjoy it.

Like the first one, this exercise is vitally important. We urge you to include it in your pleasuring repertoire.

Tactile Inventory

Here is your chance to touch yourself all over your body, *except your genitals*. Touch yourself in all kinds of ways, including pinching, scratching, light touches, firm touches, quick touches, and long or short strokes. The goals are to see what feels best, to learn to feel pleasure with a variety of strokes and pressures, and to increase your capacity to focus your attention on the places you are touching.

When we ask you to combine your touches with your full attention, we mean that we want you to isolate the area in your mind to allow it to feel as much as it can in the moment. Doing this to yourself is easier than having someone else do it to you because your own touch will not be a surprise. Nor will you feel any vulnerability. This is your time, and the goal is to experience as much pleasure as you possibly can in this moment. If you find your mind wandering, just notice it, and then put your attention back onto the sensations. Notice which parts of your body are the most sensitive and which areas prefer a light or a firm touch. Do this exercise for as long as it is fun to do. There is no time limit, minimum or maximum, and breaks are encouraged.

Try a single touch on different areas, especially the ones containing erectile tissue (nipples, lips), but also on your thighs or stomach or neck—any area that is responsive and feels good to touch. Notice whether you feel any sensation in any other part of your body, including your genitals, when you touch these spots. Remember, for now, to avoid touching the genitals.

Also try stroking some areas. Apply a little lubricant to your finger and place it on an area containing erectile tissue, such as your lips or nipples— or on any other area that you choose. First, do a single touch with lubricant. Then try different types of strokes. Try different pressures and different movements; again, this is a time to experiment.

Once you have created a connection between your clitoris or penis and different body parts, as described further below, to turn yourself on you can simply touch these sensitive areas. This will coincide with your ability to experience instant orgasm. We have done these exercises hundreds of times ourselves, and each time we may focus on a different area of the body or a different aspect of the experience. So do not think that you are just doing the same thing over and over; be creative and experiment.

⋟ Masturbation and Connections ⋞

If you have been doing these exercises in the proper order, your body will probably be very tumesced, or excited, at this point. This is what you want. In this next exercise we want you to make your genitals, specifically your clitoris or penis, the focal point. By this, we mean we want you to spend time touching the area *around* the focal point to arouse yourself through anticipation. We want you to tease yourself. You can use either touches or strokes here, whatever feels best. A light, quick stroke will usually increase your arousal. Approach the focal area and then withdraw, continuing to do so for as long as you like.

When you are ready to put your full attention on your clitoris or penis, apply some lubricant to the area in any way that feels good. You can apply it slowly, working your way toward the focal point, or quickly, so that the lubrication process does not become your primary concern. Again, we believe it is a good idea to experiment with various touches, strokes, and pressures; that is, each time you practice this exercise, do it somewhat differently.

For Women

Continue to tease yourself around your genitals, avoiding directly touching your clitoris for as long as you like. Eventually you will want to lubricate your inner lips, introitus, and perineum, and then finally move on to your clitoris. You can take your time, lingering over any area that feels especially wonderful, or you can quickly spread lubricant over the entire area. When you are ready to touch your clitoris, put a small dab of lubricant on your fingertip and pull back your hood to expose the head. Spread the lubricant over the entire head of your clitoris.

Chapter 5 details many ways to retract the clitoral hood and spread lubricant. For this exercise, however, we want you to touch your clitoris using only one type of stroke. Try a short stroke, focusing on the most sensitive part of your clitoris, wherever this is for you. To discover which part of your clitoris is the most sensitive, start by stroking all the different quadrants, one at a time. You can also try a longer stroke, moving from bottom to top on the left side, and then switch your strokes to the right side. The object is to experience as much feeling as you can and also to notice which areas feel best and which kinds of strokes you prefer—light or firm, fast or slow.

Continue, one stroke at a time, for as long as you enjoy it. At some point, start stroking yourself without pausing between strokes. This should get you going a little more intensely. You can always stop when you want to peak— that is, when you want to allow your level of arousal to decrease a little so you can take things higher with the next stroke or series of strokes (described in more detail in Chapter 7). But try to be aware of how many strokes you can feel without losing focus either mentally or physically. Do this for as long as you like, from a few seconds to many minutes. The longer you practice this part of the exercise, the more often you can take breaks and peak yourself.

Adding Connections

When your clitoris is feeling really good, we want you to add a secondary area to the equation. This can be any other part of your body; however, we recommend using an area that has erectile tissue, such as your lips (either facial or vaginal), your anus, or your nipple. Apply a little lubricant to the particular area. Hopefully, your clitoris will be engorged enough by now so that it bulges freely away from the body and you no longer have to pull the hood back.

Simultaneously stroke both your clitoris and the secondary area with the same kind of stroke. You may want to start by using a single stroke, simultaneously stroking both areas one time, then stopping for a few moments, then repeating. Do this a number of times. Then just stroke your clitoris for one stroke while removing your hand from the secondary area. For the next few repetitions, again stroke the areas at the same time. Next, stroke your secondary spot while leaving your hand off your clitoris. Then once again stroke them both. We are trying to build a connection between your clitoris and the secondary area. Be patient. Notice if you feel any sensation in the area that is *not* being touched.

After doing the single-stroke technique, try some continuous strokes, stroking both areas in-sync. Repeat the above instructions, alternately removing your hand from the secondary area and then the clitoris, but this time use continuous strokes rather than single strokes. When your hand is removed from either body part, continue the stroking motion in the air, slightly above the body.

Again, the more you practice this exercise, the more you will build a connection between your clitoris and other parts of your body. This is helpful to women who are not easily orgasmic during intercourse, as they learn to connect their labia minora and introitus to their clitoris in such a way that that when the penis is inserted they can feel more sensation and possibly reach orgasm. It is also fun to connect the lips of your mouth with your clitoris so that kissing will become that much more sensational. The lips-to-genital connection works for men as well as women, of course.

For Men

When touching yourself, you can use a video, a magazine, or a mental fantasy. Play with and almost tease your body by stroking nongenital erotic areas, such as your nipples or lips or stomach or thighs—whatever feels good. We recommend lightly stroking your inner thighs, getting close to your genitals, and then backing away. You can play with one stroke at a time, even on your thighs, and then add some continuous stroking.

We also suggest moving your lower abdomen, which is physically connected to your pubic area, up and down by pressing your hand into your body with as much pressure as feels good to you (see Figure 5 on page 37). You can alternatively use just your fingers to press into the lower abdomen and pubic area in order to find the spot and pressure that feel the best. You can use all of your fingers on one spot or find a couple of areas close to each other and press with one or two fingers at a time on one spot before releasing the pressure and pressing with two other fingers on the second spot. You might also enjoy using two hands—one on either side of your upper pubic or lower abdominal area—by pressing with both hands at the same time or by alternating between pressing and releasing. You can have fun experimenting here to find what works best for you. Note that both men and women find the lower abdominal area to be pleasurable to the touch.

Approve of all the sensations you experience, and only continue for as long as the feelings keep getting better. You may lightly brush your pubic hair with the back or front or side of your hand, or you may gently stroke your scrotal area from bottom to top. You can play with different areas around your genitals, such as your perineum, anus, and scrotum. You can use single strokes or apply different pressures—whatever feels best. By now your penis is probably erect and you are hopefully feeling much pleasure down there. Again, remember that the penis does not have to be erect to do these exercises, or even to feel pleasure.

Applying Lubricant

Put some lubricant on one finger and apply it to the part of your penis that most desires to be touched. The location and size of the area is up to you. You can do this very nimbly and gently; usually, the more trained a man becomes, the more he can enjoy a light touch. You want to feel as much as you can with every touch, including the application of the lubricant. This is another opportunity to practice the single touch, only this time using some lubricant, which can make it ever so much more pleasurable. You can then apply more lubricant to another part of your penis. You may feel tingles and actual contractions as you do this. You might already be close to orgasm merely as a result of applying the lubricant. Continue applying lubricant in small amounts until your entire penis is covered and well lubricated. I like to save the frenulum or apex (see Figure 6) for last, as it is the most sensitive part of the penis and thus serves as the focal point. A single, final touch on this exquisite area with some lubricant may bring you to a high level of arousal.

What we just described is one way to apply lubricant that is very luxurious and deliberate. You can also place a bigger batch of lubricant all over your fingers and apply it from the base of the penis to the tip in one stroke, using the hand as a kind of tube. Or you can apply the lubricant starting on a different side of your penis each time. One time you can start on the posterior side and work your way to the sensitive underneath area, or anterior side; another time you can put it on your most sensitive area first and then spread it around.

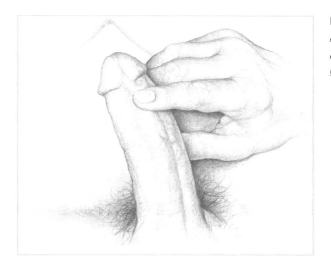

Figure 6.
*Erect penis
showing apex
(or frenulum)*

Whether you do it slowly, using a little lubricant at a time, or quickly, with a lot of lubricant, depends on how you feel at the moment. I usually prefer to start lubricating the least sensitive areas first and work my way slowly to the most sensitive ones.

There are many ways to apply lubricant, and you can ask your partner to be creative in this sensual act as well as being innovative yourself. You can always think up new ways to apply lubricant. It is all about pleasure, and as long as you are enjoying the process you will be enhancing your pleasure. Sometimes I don't feel that interested in self-pleasure, but as soon as I start touching myself with some lubricant my interest greatly increases. I know I will be in "pleasure mode" as soon as the first bit of lubricant reaches my penis. However, as soon as you catch your thoughts slipping into the future while you're doing anything, even lubricating, take a little break.

Single-Touch and Single-Stroke Masturbation

Once you have lubricated your entire penis you can start masturbating, first using one touch at a time and then using one stroke at a time. Check out different touches and strokes. Just touch yourself—aiming for as much pleasure and sensation as you can muster—and then remove your hand. Touch and stroke different parts of your penis to see where it feels best. As we have said, most men are most sensitive right below the corona, on the underside of the penis, so give yourself some single strokes there. One at a time, try some short strokes and some longer strokes, discovering how much you can feel with each kind. Play with different pressures, different speeds, and different types of strokes. Anything that you can come up with is okay as long as it feels good. Remember, give yourself only one stroke at a time for now.

Starting to Connect

Now touch the most sensitive area of your penis with one hand while you simultaneously touch a secondary area with your other hand. It may be best to choose a secondary area that contains erectile tissue, such as lips, nipples, or anus. Put some lubricant on the secondary area, too, especially when you start stroking it. Do only a single stroke or touch, and then stop. Use the same kind of touch or stroke on both areas.

Continue touching both areas a number of times, and then touch only your penis. Notice whether you feel anything at all in your secondary area, even if it is only some heat or a slight sensation. Then once again touch the two areas at the same time for a few strokes, stopping after each stroke. Next, touch only your secondary area, and see if you can feel any sensation in your penis. Don't feel bad if you feel nothing or only a little bit; it takes practice to build a good connection. Now try some single strokes on both areas at the same time and see if this increases the sensation. Then, using one stroke at a time, stroke only your penis, then both places, and then only your secondary area. Use the strokes that you found most pleasurable when you did the single-stroke masturbation exercise. Anticipate the strokes by focusing your attention on where you will be touching and stroking.

Steady Stroking

Now it is time for some steady stroking. We want you to get to a higher level of intensity so that you can possibly make a better connection. You are fully lubricated, but you can always add some more if you feel at all dry.

Use your favorite strokes. We recommend repeating reliable strokes of the same type to take you higher. We also think that using a stroke that provides a great deal of contact between hand and penis will stimulate the most nerves. That being said, you will want to experiment and check out many different kinds of strokes—from short ones to long ones, from full hand to fingertip. As long as you repeat the same stroke a number of times, you will allow yourself to go higher; as soon as you change the stroke, you will probably go down (peak) for a short time until you've repeated that stroke a number of times, too. (Peaking is one of the most important concepts in creating an EMO and is fully discussed in Chapter 7.)

Steady-Stroke Connections

We are still interested in creating connections between your penis and the rest of your body. Take a little lubricant in your free hand and select a secondary area. Repeat the same steady stroke on both areas. Do this for a while, and then remove your hand or finger from the secondary area. Keep it just above the skin while still moving your hand as if you were stroking yourself. Notice any sensation in the secondary area, and continue as long as the sensation there continues. When the sensation ends, put your hand back on the secondary area and rub the two areas in tandem again. After stroking them simultaneously for a while, take your hand off your penis and, in the air just above the penis, continue with your stroking motion. Notice if you have any sensation in your penis. As before, continue this motion until all sensation ends, and then put your hand back on your penis and stroke both areas simultaneously again. When you change the stroke on your penis, change the stroke on your secondary area. The more often you practice this exercise, the more of a connection you will build.

These activities are for your enjoyment and education. You can continue with the connections exercise, or you can do it for a while and then go back to masturbating. You can peak yourself as many times as you like, getting close to ejaculation but not going over. Experiment and have fun.

⇒ Once You've Built a Connection ⇐

Once you build a connection, you can play with your connected areas at times when touching your genitals may be inappropriate. You can touch yourself anywhere and feel more pleasure than you used to. Just think how much fun kissing can become when your lips are supersensitive. Don't worry about becoming so sensitive that you will feel too much pleasure at inappropriate times. You can always put a damper on those nerve endings by deciding when and where it's okay to feel pleasure.

If you practice these exercises regularly, when you have a sensual experience you will be amazed at how much increased sensation you feel everywhere on your body, including your genitals. A real EMO is a whole-body orgasm. If you connect up your whole body, you may experience instant pleasure at the moment when someone first touches you, no matter where they touch you. You will have better orgasms that begin right away and last longer.

The next chapter investigates how to communicate with your partner about sensual matters and how to train him or her to be the best lover possible.

CHAPTER 3

Pleasure Training

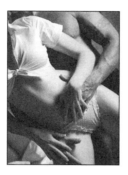

*T*he ability to use language has put human beings at the top of the food chain. It has enabled
us to be better hunters and planners, and to teach
and question our fellow humans. We have learned many
things from our ancestors, including both good and bad
ideas—"good" and "bad" being concepts that actually
depend on one's point of view. Nothing is inherently good
or bad on its own; whether we label it so depends on our
goals in relation to the event or action. Rain in itself is
neither good nor bad; the farmer who needs rain to grow
crops will consider it good, and the baseball fan who
wants to go to the game will view it as bad.

⋙ Inheriting Information ⋘

The passing on of information about how to do anything is language dependent, including making war (good or bad?), collecting taxes (good or bad?), and increasing crop yield (good or bad?). Language affects every aspect of our lives. We obviously have some basic instincts, such as those for eating and procreating. Eating may be instinctual, but creating a gourmet meal is not, and the information about how to do so can only be passed on using some kind of language skills. Knowledge about procreation has been passed on without much use of language. It is obvious that human beings are good at procreating. What is less obvious is that procreation and creating pleasure are usually two different functions, and we have virtually ignored the possibilities inherent in the latter, despite our advanced language skills. The analogy between eating to survive and preparing gourmet meals applies here and highlights this difference. It may not even be that the ability to create pleasure has been ignored so much as it hasn't been fully studied. For whatever set of reasons, most of the information about sex that has been passed down is either negative or misleading. (Some may disagree with this assessment, of course, depending on their goals, but our goal is to create more pleasure.)

It does seem unusual that there is so much negativity about sex in our society. We have been conditioned to regard as evil and sinful something as basic and enjoyable as pleasuring the human body. For most of our history we have been kept in the dark about how to produce great tactile and sensual pleasures. Most of us have been made to believe that we are not supposed to talk while having sex. Almost all, if not all, the people we know, including our students, complain about having difficulty talking when experiencing or producing pleasure. Here we are, the animal with the greatest ability to communicate, and we are largely unable to express ourselves while experiencing the highest level of pleasure that is available to us.

Perhaps the biggest misfortune arising from this state of affairs is the inability to acknowledge the wonder and delight of a sensual experience. This lack of appreciation, this deficiency of approval of how good you feel, is a fast way to ruin the experience. It's a good way to put the kibosh on what could be a fantastic time. So while we are supposedly trying to pleasure our partners, we seldom feel comfortable acknowledge the fun we are having, and the usual human doubt creeps in. Besides taking our attention off the pleasure prize, this doubt often turns into some form of anger, reducing the level of intimacy that could have been built. It may be true that some people moan and groan and grunt to express their pleasure, which is fine. However, being that we have such wonderful language abilities, there can be a whole lot more communication within the sexual relationship—which could lead to further intimacy, a better understanding of how to pleasure your partner, and just more love for one another.

Communication about sensual matters is also lacking culturally. Until recently in our Western civilization such information was not transmitted via any method—not through the spoken or written word, and not through visual or aural means. Some ancient societies, such as the Indians, who wrote the *Kama Sutra*, passed on their sensual knowledge, but modern Eastern civilizations are puritanical in their views about sex. Some Pacific Island communities may have escaped this negative cultural conditioning, but they have not produced any great body of work that one can refer to in order to learn about pleasure. Obviously, some modern societies are more open, sexually speaking, than others, yet all are lagging behind what is possible. However, this has begun to change thanks to some trailblazers in America, such as Dr. Vic Baranco.

In our earlier books we included sections about communicating in bed. This simple idea is so vital to a great sex life that we have included it again in this book, with, of course, some new and additional information, specifically on the possibility of having instant orgasms. Note that we divide communication into two categories: training your partner to give you pleasure (that is, training from the position of pleasure recipient), and training your partner to receive pleasure (training from the position of pleasure giver).

Some people may find the word "training" offensive. They can use other words, such as teaching, coaching, instructing, or whatever they like. The result will be the same: a partner who is well versed in how to give and receive extreme pleasure. The best way to train someone is to include lots of positive acknowledgment and words of encouragement. The more appreciation you show, the more willing your partner will be to create pleasure with you, and the more confident you will both be as lovers.

Training Your Partner to Give You Pleasure

The ability to receive pleasure will vary in everyone and even in the same person at different times. This can be due to past conditioning, what is happening in the person's life at the moment, and a host of other factors. The ability to communicate one's pleasure also depends on one's conditioning and on how much training he or she has had in this practice. Anyone who really desires to experience more pleasure can increase their communication skills. When being touched for sensual pleasure there is always something about the touch or the situation that is positive. The person receiving the touch can truthfully find something they like about the sensual stimulation and can verbally acknowledge it. With more practice and conscious effort, this noticing and truthful approval of positive sensations will become easier and easier.

In the previous chapter we explored the first ingredient in improving the sensual relationship: learning how, where, and when to give yourself pleasure so that you understand more about your own body. The next ingredient is relaying this information to your partner—specifically, letting your partner know exactly how well he or she is addressing your pleasure.

Hopefully you have studied and practiced the activities described in the last chapter so that you have some knowledge about what you like and where you like it. If you and your partner are willing to explore the wide range of pleasurable touches, you can learn together what feels best. If your partner is willing, before they touch you, you can show them how you like to be touched by demonstrating on yourself. Some people have an aversion to doing this; if so, this section outlines additional ways to get your partner to touch you precisely how you want them to.

Here are the basics: Before giving your partner any instructions, first always make sure to give him or her some verbal acknowledgments. Again, the more positive feedback you give your partner, the more fun they will have giving you pleasure—and that begins before they even touch you. (In fact, the more you approve of and appreciate what is happening in all areas of your life, in bed or anywhere else, the more fun you will be to spend time with, and the more fun you will have.)

Talking also produces two more positive effects: It keeps you in present time, preventing your mind from wandering, and it allows you to receive even more pleasure by letting you fully absorb (or "swallow") the pleasure you have been given so far. Finally, by frequently acknowledging the wonderful sensations you're experiencing, you will be in a good place to make requests of your partner to change what he or she is doing. We discuss these benefits in more detail in the next chapter.

As soon as you give an instruction and your partner fulfills the request, no matter how seemingly small or simple, let them know that they have succeeded. Perhaps they have only lightened the pressure of their touch in response to your request; still, let them know that they are winning and doing well. Then, if you want even less pressure, ask again. Once they succeed, again let them know that they are doing better. Do not stop asking for what you want until your partner is doing it exactly the way you want it.

Always be sure to verbalize some positive acknowledgments before making the next request. It is more fun for your partner to do your bidding when they know how much fun you are having. Hopefully you are having a lot of fun. However, even if you're having only a little bit of pleasure and fun, you can always find something in the experience to approve of. It could be as basic as simply appreciating the fact that you are in bed together and doing an exercise. As we've said, the more you practice communicating positive feelings, the easier it will become to notice them and report them to your partner.

Give only one instruction at a time; for instance, it is not a good idea to ask for more pressure and more speed at the same time. First, get either the pressure or speed exactly where you want it, and then get the other factor dialed in. Giving too many instructions at once will only confuse your partner, causing him or her to feel inadequate.

We have taught entire courses where the goals were to learn to acknowledge positive sensations and to keep asking for what was wanted. We often have students start by rubbing on a part of the pleasure recipient's body other than the genitals so that the recipient gets accustomed to talking while receiving pleasure. Once they learn how to talk while being pleasured on their thigh, for example, they can graduate to being stimulated genitally while verbalizing approval and asking for what they want.

If you forget to approve of your partner before or after asking for a change, do not fret; just approve at the next chance you have and go on from there. Sometimes you may not know exactly what change you would like, yet you know you want something different. In this case you can experiment. Ask for something, verbalize your approval, and if it is not what you wanted ask for something else. It is best to approve of any effort to fulfill your request as soon as it is made. The longer you wait between action and approval, the less effective the training. It is also fine to ask for a break. During the break you can talk about and approve of what has occurred; then when your partner starts touching you again, either when you direct them to or on their own initiative, you will be ready for more pleasure.

Again, because it is difficult for many people to talk while having a sexual experience, we think that starting with body parts other than the genitals is a great learning tool.

Three-Step Process

So, to recap, we're talking about a three-step process:

1. Say one nice thing.
2. Ask for something.
3. Verbally reward the effort.

Repeat this sequence again and again.

The following are examples of things you can say:

* *"Wow that feels great."*
* *"I love the way you touch me."*
* *"You have great hands."*
* *"Will you use a lighter/heavier touch? Yes, that's even better."*
* *"Keep doing that."*
* *"Yes! Yes!"*
* *"You got it just right."*

So now you are in a credit situation. If you want something different, your partner will be in a great position to hear your request and do your bidding.

Training Your Partner
to Give You an Instant Orgasm

In order to practice feeling orgasmic pleasure on the first stroke, explain to your partner, before they even begin touching you, what you would like to have happen,. Tell your partner that you are learning to feel as much as you can from the very first stroke. Ask your partner to touch you with one stroke, and then to remove their hand, and then to repeat the single-stroke action over and over. You can even tell them to put their hand close to the skin without touching it to see if you can feel anything. Try using any of the exercises described in Chapter 2. Explain the activity to your partner, and then have your partner do it to you.

Remember to start by giving your partner some acknowledgments; for example, "Playing this game with you is fun," or "I am so glad we are doing this," or "You have such nice hands." Then when they touch you, you can say, "Oh, that feels great," and so on. Throughout the session, use the three-step process described above.

This method of training through positive communication works in any situation, not just in bed, but it may take some getting used to. We aren't accustomed to verbalizing much approval and appreciation, even in everyday activities.

⇒ Training Your Partner to ⇐ Receive Pleasure

The person giving the pleasure has to learn to take control of their partner's nervous system. This requires confidence that they know what to do. Start by setting up the space so that all towels, lubricants, pillows, etc., are in place. To find out what your partner would like for you to do to them, it is best to ask specific questions, which we discuss below. You also must make your partner feel like they are being taken care of; this will help them relax and feel safe enough to surrender. Therefore, it is useful to inform your partner of what you are going to do next and to report all activities and sensations you notice that could affect your partner's level of relaxation.

Always let your partner know what is going to happen next—even before putting your hands on your partner's body, before relocating your hands, and before removing them. For example, if the phone rings you can take charge by announcing that you will let the answering machine pick up. A thorough giver of pleasure will often make sure that the phone's ringer is turned off before beginning the sensual activity.

Sometimes when a woman who has never rubbed on me before is not talking much, I may start to wonder what she is doing, whether she knows how to make me squirt, or if she even wants to. If she were to say that she is having fun playing with my penis and that she is not ready to squirt me just yet, and when she is she will let me know, this would allow me to surrender more to her manipulations, which would bring me far more pleasure than if she did not talk. Whether you're pleasuring a woman or a man, merely by saying a few simple words you can take more control of the situation than by saying little or nothing.

It is sensual and fun to report to your partner all the signs of pleasure and orgasm that you notice happening in his or her body. Sometimes the genitals of the person giving pleasure will feel wonderful even though they are using their hands. (The same is true if you are giving oral sex, but you will have difficulty expressing yourself with your mouth occupied!) Let your partner know about this pleasure you're feeling, *unless* you think it would detract from their sense of pleasure and relaxation. I know for myself that when a woman who is pleasuring me with her hands tells me that she feels intense sensations in her pussy, it increases my own pleasure. So when I am stroking a woman, if my penis is getting erect or leaking semen I will usually tell her. Again, if you believe this information would make her feel uncomfortable or threatened, you can always tell her later or not at all. In the next chapter we go into more detail about reporting on your own pleasure and noting the signs of pleasure you observe in your partner.

Questions to Ask

To determine your partner's desires, the best types of questions to ask are simple ones that he or she can answer with either a yes or a no. You do not want your partner to have to think too much while they are supposed to be at total effect (that is, completely immersed in the sensations they are feeling), so a question like "What do you want next?" or "Tell me how you feel," or "How am I doing?"—any type of essay question—is not part of the training.

Furthermore, the yes-or-no question has to be presented so that the answer given will be acceptable to you. Questions like "Would you like it harder?" or "Would you like it lighter?" are satisfactory, but questions like "Do you like this?" or "Does this feel good?" potentially set you up to lose. If it does not feel good and your partner says so, you will feel a loss. Additionally, if they say yes, they could be lying because they don't want to hurt your feelings. Only ask questions to which the answer, yes or no, will make no difference in how you are feeling emotionally.

Once you get a yes to a question you've asked, go ahead and perform the action involved, *using small increments*. You do not want to ask your partner if they would like more pressure and then give them a lot more pressure. Give them a little more pressure, and then ask again if they would like even more pressure. Keep asking simple questions and responding to your partner's answers until you have it just right.

Other questions that are easy to ask and are helpful can be about direction, speed, or insertion, for instance:

* *"Would you like it more to the left?"*
* *"More to the right?"*
* *"Would you like it higher?"*
* *"Lower?"*
* *"Would you like a shorter stroke?"*
* *"A longer stroke?"*
* *"A faster stroke?"*
* *"A slower stroke?"*
* *"A deeper stroke?"*
* *"Would you like me to stroke you more under the hood?"*
* *"Would you like more lubricant?"*
* *"Would you like to take a break?"*

If you are giving pleasure to a male partner you can ask:

* *"Do you want me to use one hand?"*

* *"Two hands?"*

* *"Do you want your testicles played with?"*

* *"How about under the testicles?"*

* *"Do you want more pressure under your testicles?"*

A pleasure recipient of either sex can be asked if they want their anus played with. Whatever activity you can think of that you would enjoy doing, go ahead and ask. In this way you will discover what your partner likes—and you may even create some new experiences that they will learn to enjoy.

Again, in our classes we sometimes have people ask these kinds of questions while stroking on an area other than the genitals. This helps them learn how to ask the right questions in a situation that is less charged or exciting than touching the genitals. They can first learn how to talk and ask the right questions and then graduate to genitals.

Training Your Partner
to Receive an Instant Orgasm

Here are some pointers for training your partner to have an instant orgasm:

◆ Discuss in advance what you will be doing.

◆ Tell them where you will be touching them.

◆ Tell them how many strokes you will be using (preferably one to start with).

◆ After giving the initial stroke(s), use yes-or-no questions to determine if they would like a longer stroke or a shorter one, or more pressure, or less pressure, or more to the left, or more to the right, etc.

◆ Continue giving strokes, asking yes-or-no questions, and adjusting as necessary.

◆ Throughout the process, describe aloud any response you notice in your partner's body and also in your own.

Also try placing your finger directly above the clitoris, without touching it, and then ask if they can feel your finger.

If you're giving pleasure to a man, follow the same guidelines. Give him one stroke, then ask if he would like more than one, and then give him two strokes, and so on.

Remember that people will pay more attention to what they are feeling when they are not being stroked over and over with the aim of getting somewhere. They will learn to feel more from the first stroke. The communication that goes with this technique is important so that the person receiving the pleasure is not in suspense about what is happening and can respond to the requests given them (see below for more on making requests of the pleasure recipient).

Consult Chapter 2, including the connections exercises, for many different ideas on how to touch a woman or a man. Again, this is a time to experiment and find out what your partner prefers. Besides the ways of touching that we've outlined in this book, explore any idea that pops into your head. Using your new communication tools, first ask your partner if she or he would like you to touch her or him in that way.

Putting the Training Together: Receiver and Giver

For the training to work, it takes only one person to either request what they want or to ask the right questions. The training can therefore be done from either side—from the position of receiver or giver of pleasure. However, when both partners are communicating at the same time, the training will become more effective and will happen faster. The person receiving the pleasure will be giving lots of acknowledgments and requesting exactly what they want, and the person giving the pleasure will take control by asking simple yes-or-no questions. The result will be a more precise and quicker discovery of exactly how to gratify the person who is being pleasured.

This is an excellent way to practice feeling that first stroke by limiting the number of strokes requested each time, as described above. The person giving the pleasure wants to learn to take control and will decide how many strokes to use and where to begin, preferably using only one and by placing their hand near but not touching the clitoris or penis. Then the person receiving can respond by expressing appreciation and perhaps asking for a specific stroke.

The back-and-forth conversation will make the experience more fun and fulfilling, and both partners will learn from it. At some point you will both be able to feel more on the first stroke, and hopefully your partner will be trained to touch you just the way you want to be touched. This means that after a while you will no longer have to put so much effort into training; you can just let your partner take control of your nervous system. It does *not* mean that you can stop appreciating and approving of your partner; this is as important as ever, especially for you and also somewhat for your partner. Likewise, as the pleasure giver, once you are trained with a specific partner you may no longer have to ask as many yes-or-no questions; however, you still want to take control by letting them know what is happening in their body. Also, continue reporting all signs of pleasure in your own body.

⮞ Requests, Suggestions, Commands ⮜

To give immense pleasure to another person you must pay conscious and continual attention to your communication skills. As we have stated, in order for the person receiving pleasure to fully surrender, the person giving the pleasure must assume control—or at least the semblance of control. Here's what we mean by "semblance of control": The pleasure giver, even though they are the one in control, is still responding to the pleasure recipient. Every orgasm is really determined by the individual who is receiving the attention. As the pleasure giver, we can only *suggest* that the recipient allow more pleasure; we cannot force them to. Yet this gives us a great deal of leeway and allows us to play with the one being pleasured to a large degree. You have to know whom you are dealing with to implement the best strategy for applying control. What is the best way to talk to this person? What kind of influence will they respond to? Some people really like it when you tell them rather forcefully what to do, while others prefer a more gentle, coaxing approach. If you talk harshly to someone who resists and resents this kind of speech, then you will fail at giving them more pleasure. Conversely, if you speak gently to someone who likes rough talk, again you will have missed an opportunity.

Most people like to hear that they are doing well and are being fun, so as long as you can truthfully acknowledge anything positive you've noticed, it is a good idea to do so. On the other hand, if your partner is being resistant or is obviously not being, or having, fun, it is time to talk, ask questions, and get to the bottom of the problem.

When we work with a student, we want to produce the most pleasure in her body that we can. This often requires that we give her suggestions on how to do better. We may ask her to feel more, to take it higher, to give it up, to relax her body—whatever we think will work. As soon as she responds, we reward her efforts by acknowledging that we can sense her arousal increasing and by telling her that she is doing well. Before we even start touching her we inform her that we may use some suggestions or commands and that in response she really does not have to do anything; her body will respond correctly by simply hearing the word "Relax" or "Take it higher." We emphasize that she must not feel bad if we ask her to go higher, as it does not mean that she is not doing well, only that we want to take her to the next level.

⇒ More Instant-Orgasm Training ⇐

When teaching a woman student to get off instantly, we use certain directives. We may tell her in advance that we will be using many short cycles to enable her to feel more from the first stoke. We may start with parts of her body other than her genitals—maybe her thigh or nipple or the lips of her mouth. We may touch her only briefly or perhaps give her continual strokes. We may move our touches from place to place on her body, always saying in advance where we are going to touch next.

We may then, without touching her, hold our hand just above her genitals, getting close to the clitoris, and ask her to feel the focus and attention on her clitoris. We may proceed to touching her inner labia, perineum, or mons pubis (see Figure 1 on page 33), inform her what is coming next, and ask her to put her full attention on that area.

When eventually we do touch the genitals, avoiding the clitoris and clitoral hood for now, it may be with a finger, or a lightly applied knuckle, or a whole palm. We may use a single stroke or stay in one spot and employ different degrees of pressure, continually communicating what we are doing and asking the student to feel that area. Then we may get out the lubricant, again telling her what we are doing, and, using a finger, place some lubricant on her erectile tissue, such as the perineum or the labia minora. Or we may return to the nipple, playing with the application of lubricant there. The whole time, we ask her to feel the area that we are lubricating.

Once we have applied lubricant all over her genitals—still avoiding the clitoris and clitoral hood—we may give her some additional strokes on the labia or other parts of her genitals, each time asking her to feel the stroke to the best of her ability. Now we move toward the clitoris. I sometimes like to use what we call the "Michael Douglas" stroke (see Figure 7), slowly approaching the clitoral shaft with the pad of my index finger and asking her to feel my finger as it gets closer and closer to her clitoris. (We call it the Michael Douglas stroke because it reminds us of how the actor, in some of his racier movies, would press women up against the wall during sex. He used his whole body and was acting out intercourse, while we use a finger against the base of the clitoris. We will describe this stroke and others in further detail in the next few chapters.)

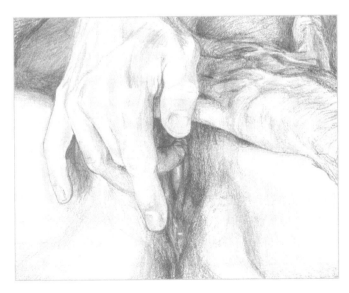

Figure 7. _Pressing against the clitoral shaft, or the "Michael Douglas" stroke_

I tell her that I am approaching her clitoris—that I am almost there. I ask her again to feel me—and there is often a fairly strong orgasmic contraction when the finger does finally contact the clitoral shaft. It's almost as if the entire clitoris is reaching out toward my finger. I tell her that was a nice contraction, I back off, and then I restart the slow progression toward the clitoris, again continually describing what is happening and what I expect from her.

As you can see, what we're doing is combining words and touches to train the student to eagerly anticipate, to practically beg for, the very first clitoral touch, thereby greatly increasing the orgasmic sensation she will feel when we finally do get there.

➣ Talking while Pleasuring a Man ➢

A woman can play with a man's penis in a similar fashion, describing what she is doing and telling him to focus his attention on her touch. Again, it is important to size up your partner to determine what kind of communication works best. In the same way that women appreciate confident givers of pleasure, many men like it when their partners are sure of themselves and communicate accordingly. When a woman is giving me pleasure I prefer that she take control of my body and the situation, allowing me just to lie back and feel and occasionally acknowledge my pleasure. Of course, most people have to first be trained to touch you where and how you want them to. Once a woman is trained, I know that I like for her to touch my penis as if she owned it and knew what she was doing, and also to communicate with me that she is thoroughly enjoying what she is doing.

She can tell me to feel more. She can say that she is going to go faster or use more pressure or whatever. In this way I do not have to worry about whether she knows what she is doing. She can tell me that she knows she could squirt me in five strokes but is not going to, or that she is going for the final peak now. She can say things like "I've got you," "You are under my control," and "I can take you whenever or wherever I want to."

A woman can find out if her guy is a leg man or a breast man or a butt man. She can play with fantasy and tell him that she is squeezing his penis between her thighs or against her breast or, if he likes feet, that she is rubbing his penis between her feet and calves. One time, while a woman was giving me pleasure, she said that she was going to rub my cock between her thighs and finish me off with her calves. This really made me go higher in intensity and enjoyment. Whatever it is that turns your man on can be used to produce more fun and pleasure.

If she thinks she would enjoy it, she can even do these things while she talks about them, such as rubbing his penis with her calves or thighs or breast. Sometimes the mere suggestion of something is as good as or even better than the activity itself. The fantasy may be difficult to actually perform, may be impractical, or may be less fun than the suggestion. For instance, if a woman has razor stubble on her legs, the act of rubbing her guy's penis between her calves will not be as pleasurable for him as the suggestion of doing so.

Through the power of imagination, you can even bring other people into the sex act without having their actual bodies in the room. Sometimes when Vera is pleasuring me she may bring up the name of some other woman whom she knows I find sexy and talk about having that woman do things to me.

Words are incredibly powerful tools, and boosting one's skill at communicating in bed will make the difference between being an okay lover and being a fantastic one.

⇒ Asking for What You Want ⇐

It is so important to know what you like and to have the communication skills to ask for it to be done exactly the way you want it. You can enjoy surrendering yourself to the whim of your partner and letting them do as they see fit, but lovemaking is even more fun for everyone if partners can express their specific desires. For instance, if you feel extra sensitive today, let your partner know. If you want to be touched faster or slower or harder or whatever, even if you have already trained your partner, ask for it in a polite way, as we outlined in the sections on training your partner.

Here's a simple example of the importance of clearly communicating one's desires instead of beating around the bush. Vera and I were coming home from a long day's outing, and she asked if I wanted to go upstairs first or get the mail. I said I'd like to go upstairs first. Then she said she wanted to get the mail first, which caused me to feel in some small way like I'd lost. Instead of asking me what I wanted and then overriding it, she could have just said that she wanted to get the mail before going upstairs, allowing us both to win. This situation didn't carry much charge, of course, but it's that much more important to ask for what you want in a sensual or sexual setting because of the heightened vulnerability many of us feel when we're in bed. Our conditioning against doing so is quite strong, so being able to speak one's desires straight-forwardly and with ease takes deliberate practice and intention. It is not easy to do in everyday life, and it is even more difficult to do in bed.

⤏ Connecting the Brain to the Genitals ⤸

We recently met a very attractive and appealing woman in her late thirties. She told us she'd been easily pleasured in her youth but a few years ago had a boyfriend who used way too much pressure during oral sex. It hurt a lot and caused severe bruising. The experience caused her such severe mental trauma that she didn't want to engage in any kind of sexual activity for over three years. The boyfriend obviously did not know what he was doing to her, and she did not tell him to stop as soon as it felt bad, which was right away. As a result, her resistance caused her to turn off her brain from feeling almost any pleasure in her genitals.

She could have avoided this whole negative experience if she'd had more societal encouragement and conditioning to communicate properly in bed. She could have told him as soon as he started that she would like it a lot lighter. Before she came to see us, she had not told anyone about this episode except her doctor, who informed her that he had seen much worse. In our work with her, we heaped lots of approval on her and communicated about what we were doing at every step. Eventually, this made her feel safe and relaxed so that she was once again able to feel pleasure in her genitals. It took a while. At first there was not a complete connection between how much pleasure her genitals were having (as evidenced by their physical response) and the pleasure she al-lowed herself to feel in her mind. But after a few more sessions she was able to feel a lot of pleasure in both her genitals and her brain.

We have noticed this resistance in other people—that is, a disconnect between the amount of pleasure the brain and the genitals are feeling. It is as though all the sensation is somehow not getting through; there is a road-block separating body from brain. By continually approving of the physical reactions we notice, pointing out the individual contractions as they happen, and getting the student to feel increasingly comfortable with this new type of sensation, we usually succeed in fully connecting their brain with their genitals. In the next chapter we will describe a number of other resistances to pleasure that we have encountered and the best ways we have found to handle them.

∼

By following the directions in this chapter you will become proficient in your ability to communicate well during any sensual act. By practicing acknowledgment and approval in all aspects of your life, in and out of bed, your capacity for increased fun and pleasure will manifest. The next chapters focus on specific techniques for pleasuring one's partner, how to feel more pleasure oneself, and how to overcome resistances. If you practice these skills, you will become an exceptional lover.

CHAPTER 4

Partnered Pleasure

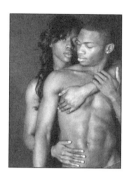

*N*ow that you know how to pleasure yourself and how to train your partner, it is time to go into greater detail about communication skills, about giving and receiving pleasure, and about how to cause your partner to feel even more intensely, especially at the beginning of a sensual experience. The more intensely a person can feel at that very first stroke, the more they will feel as a result of all the strokes that come after.

For the most part, this chapter discusses techniques that can be used with a partner of either gender, but we will let you know when the information applies specifically to one or the other. The chapter expands on the importance of using approval and verbal acknowledgment to experience the most pleasure possible. It outlines some of our strategies for facilitating increased pleasure in the recipient. It describes what to do when confronting a person's resistance to pleasure, even if that person is verbally saying yes.

Keep in mind that resistances are a part of the pleasuring game. They can actually create more pleasure if handled in a fun and appropriate way. Resistances are comparable to obstacles met on the path to a goal. Having to overcome problems or difficulties increases the value you place on the attainment of your goal, and having to creatively overcome a partner's resistances to pleasure enhances the enjoyment of the sensual encounter.

Pleasuring a Partner: Some Basics

Whether it is the first stroke or the thousandth, you have to know whether or not a person, especially a woman, really wants your hands on their body. You have to trust your integrity and your gut feelings, and if there is any doubt about whether or not to proceed, it is best not to. Pause, take a break, and talk a bit more. Ask questions, for example, "Have you had enough?" or "Would you like more strokes?"

Another very important aspect of pleasuring someone is to make sure that you, the pleasure giver, are enjoying what you are doing. If you are not relishing your own handiwork you will convey that message to the other person. As counterintuitive as it may sound, you must touch her or him for your own pleasure; you must make your hand or fingers or lips or whatever you are touching with feel as good as possible with each stroke or caress. You have to touch your partner for your own selfish reasons. If you do that, the person you are pleasuring will not feel that they owe you anything in return. This will allow them to relax and surrender to the pleasure.

Surrendering one's nervous system is a key ingredient in having an IO or an EMO. Anything you do to facilitate surrender in your partner will be well worth your while. If they think they have to give something back—that because you rubbed their back they have to rub yours—it will lessen their pleasure and their ability to surrender. This does not mean they can't reciprocate if they want to, only that they do not *have* to. There is a big difference between the two, and the sooner you understand this, the more fun you will have.

If you are with a new or fairly new partner it may be a good idea to let them know that you love giving pleasure and that they are under no obligation to give anything back in return. The best way to demonstrate this is by really enjoying what you are doing to them. They will certainly be able to sense it if that's the case. Sometimes we advise our male students to leave their clothes on when pleasuring a woman, even a close partner, so that she will know he has no ulterior motives. The least he can do is to ask her preference about this. (In contrast, because males are so visually oriented, when a woman is pleasuring a man it is often a good idea for her to remove at least some of her clothes to enhance his view.)

You want to create a safe and pleasant environment for your pleasure activities. Whether it is the bed or a soft rug in front of the fireplace, take time to set up the space so you have all your accessories nearby, such as extra pillows, lubricant, and something to drink. Follow the guidelines that we provided in the self-pleasuring exercises in Chapter 2. The goal is to make sure that both you and your partner are very comfortable. As part of creating the atmosphere, it is a good idea beforehand to talk about the impending experience. This should help to get your partner into the mood and to accept the feeling of being attended to.

More on the Importance of Acknowledgment

When being pleasured, it is best to be at total effect. Basically, this means we want you just to lie there and feel. There is one important exception to this rule and that is to acknowledge any and all positive feelings you experience, a topic we introduced in the previous chapter and wish to expand on here. This is one of the most difficult yet important parts of learning how to receive great pleasure. It is difficult because, as we have said, we have been conditioned by our society to avoid talking during a sensual encounter. It is important for at least three reasons:

1. To Stay in Present Time

The first reason to acknowledge your pleasure is because it keeps you in present time. The more you can connect the pleasure in your genitals with your brain by speaking appreciative words, the more you will be focused on the present moment rather than drifting into your head and leaving the scene.

Speak up and acknowledge pleasant sensations, yet do so without thinking too hard about what to say. Simple statements such as "That feels great," or "Yes," or "Keep doing that" are all that is necessary. Once a person learns to speak easily when being pleasured, they can get a little more creative. Comments like "That light stroke on my clitoris is so fine," or "Your finger is on the perfect spot," or "I can feel the electricity go down my leg to my foot" are some examples.

As we said in the previous chapter, the pleasure giver is also well advised to acknowledge the pleasure they are experiencing. Doing so will help to keep them in present time and prevent them from drifting into their heads. Say things like "Your contractions feel so good against my thumb" or "Your pussy feels so delicious." You can also report on what you notice in the body of the person you are pleasuring. Try statements like "Your face and neck are fully flushed and look beautiful" or "I just felt your clitoris become harder and more engorged." This sort of verbal appreciation works for any person of either sex while receiving or giving pleasure.

2. To Create More Pleasure

A second reason for verbally acknowledging the pleasure you are receiving is that the act of appreciating enables you to finish a cycle and go on to the next level. We call this part of the pleasure cycle "swallowing." It is a form of consumption that is often overlooked, which causes more problems than anything else in life, especially during sensual activity. If you were to eat without swallowing, you would find it impossible to keep eating. It is equally important to chew the food properly. Sensually speaking, this means you want to taste and relish each morsel, and it applies to receiving the next great stroke as much as it does to eating.

So by verbally acknowledging your pleasure, you are actually committing a selfish act—in a good way, of course. People who are too angry or lazy or whatever to communicate their positive feelings actually hurt themselves the most. They cannot go to the next pleasurable level, and, in fact, actually create a downward cycle leading to decreased pleasure.

3. To Keep Your Partner Interested

A third reason to verbally acknowledge your pleasure is to communicate that you are enjoying the experience so the person giving you pleasure knows they are succeeding. Most men, especially, have some doubt about their ability to produce pleasure in a woman's body. Your reassurance that you like what your partner is doing will make him or her want to continue doing it, and they will feel good about themselves and about you. Men are success junkies, and a little approval will make them want to give you even more pleasure. If you fail to show much approval or to communicate your appreciation for their actions, they will doubt that you are enjoying yourself and will probably want to stop—even if you are secretly loving the experience. Moaning and making sounds is sometimes effective, but it is much better to use specific words.

Men can have a tendency to overproduce. A man has to learn to end the action or take a break before the person he is pleasuring stops wanting more. We will describe how to do this in Chapter 7, "The Pleasure of Peaking."

A lack of acknowledgment is probably the single most problematic thing in lovemaking and in relationships in general. If more couples verbally acknowledged and appreciated each other, there would be far fewer divorces. A doubt that your partner appreciates you can and often does turn into some form of anger, which often shows up as an avoidance of confrontation or a lack of attention to the relationship. Things will not get any better until at least one person starts to talk. Again, by acknowledging the fun you are receiving you reward your partner, which will ultimately benefit you, too.

➤ Addressing a Negative Occurrence ⇐

Of course, sometimes a negative occurrence has to be addressed, a topic we touched on in the previous chapter and that deserves another mention here. During our sessions with students, we ask them to let us know right away if there's anything they want to change. If they experience any negative feelings or physical discomfort we want them to speak up immediately instead of hoping the situation will magically take care of itself. Whenever possible, it is best to use the three-step training cycle (positive acknowledgment—request for change—positive acknowledgment) to address any negative concerns. However, if something is really injurious or harmful we would hope the person would speak up quickly. A person who is feeling negative, for whatever reason, will have little attention left for pleasure.

⇒ Dealing with the Verbally Challenged ⇐

If during a sensual session the pleasure recipient shows resistance by failing to verbally approve of the experience, there are a number of things the pleasure giver can do. The most reliable is to stop touching the person right away. Tell them that you would love to give them pleasure and that you will if they show some kind of acknowledgment or appreciation. Let them know that when they do not communicate their pleasure, you are unsure if they like what they are getting, which makes it less fun to try to pleasure them. If you address this issue before beginning the experience, then while you are pleasuring them you can remind them to speak up, and they will know why and what to do and will not become surprised and/or hurt.

A reverse-psychology trick we sometimes employ is to tell a student who is verbally challenged that for the next peak we forbid them to do any kind of acknowledging. We say we want them to be totally quiet until we tell them they can acknowledge again. We continue to do this, or we switch back and forth between voice-off and voice-on, changing the rule with each peak. A third method is for the pleasure giver to do all the verbal acknowledging for both parties. You can inform the pleasure recipient that they do not have to say anything, although they can if they so desire at any time, and that you will do the talking for both. The recipient will likely want to start talking if doing so seems fun, especially if they do not have to.

⇒ Feel the Heat ⇐

Here's a preliminary activity that will greatly intensify your first touch on your partner's body, enhancing the instantly orgasmic sensations. After a woman student has lain down, or sometimes when she is still standing, I may hold my hand over her genitals and ask if she can feel the warmth emanating from her genitals to my hand. If I feel heat coming from her genitals, I point it out to her. If I do not feel any heat, I may instruct her to send some heat down to her genitals or "pussy."

While still not touching her, I may place my hand above her throat, which is a place where sexual heat can get stuck, and ask her to direct that heat down to her genitals by focusing her attention. I then slowly lower my hand toward her genitals, moving past her breasts and belly, asking her to follow my hand with her heat.

This almost always works to some extent, and I reward her by telling her that I can feel more heat now emanating from her genitals. You can repeat the process if you want an even greater result. This sort of activity helps a person increase the feeling in their body and helps them shift their attention to where you want it to be.

⇒ Point-and-Feel Orgasm ⇐

Before getting to the bed, or maybe after the heat demonstration, I may point to a woman's clitoris and instruct her to feel my intention. Intention is the power to manifest a desire. During this activity, it is generally a good idea to tell her in advance of each step what you are going to do next, as surprises usually bring a person down. If you point to her clitoris, do it with a lot of intention and focus. Most women will admit that they feel something, but some women who aren't used to feeling much sensation will deny any feeling. Depending on how she responds to you and on how you feel, you can determine whether to continue or stop, to back off or go full steam ahead.

We have used this technique a number of times in our sensuality classes, where everyone is seated and fully clothed, and it almost always get a positive response from the woman selected. First we tell her to uncross her legs. Then, using a lot of intention, we point an index finger directly at her clitoris and ask her to feel the attention there. You can sense the excitement in the room increase. This may be the first time she has been able to feel a reaction in her genitals without contact. She will often admit to feeling contractions and a lot of pleasure there, the first signs of an instant orgasm. You may notice her face flushing, and you may experience a tingle and even an erection in your own genitals when she feels the pleasure of her clitoris. Then stop pointing. She will feel less sensation and you can sense the excitement abating. We ask the students to notice how we were able to control the whole room's level of excitement without any touching.

A man who wishes to use techniques like this that can have a strong effect on a woman must be confident in his skills. Attempting these activities without being skillful at pleasuring a woman can result in her becoming agitated rather than turned on. We do not recommend that a novice in pleasure production try the "point-and-feel" orgasm until he has gained some certainty about his abilities. It is so important for a man to learn about pleasuring others. The art of giving pleasure is both a serious and a fun educational pursuit. It will take time and lots of practice; reading books such as this one or taking a class will benefit a man greatly. Unfortunately, men are generally expected to know about sexual matters innately, and it is not easy for a man to admit that he is no sexpert. Many a man thinks that all he has to do is stick it in, and the woman will feel as much pleasure as he does. If you are a man, it will be a positive sign to a woman that you are reading this book.

⋙ Performance Anxiety ⋘

For many a woman new to IO or EMO, we have found that it is all fun and pleasure while playing and teasing around her genital area, but once the pleasure giver puts a finger directly on her clitoris she turns off the sensation. If you sense this happening, immediately tell her that you are going to remove your hands from her body, and then do so. Let her know in whatever words you wish what fantastic sensations you felt in yourself and noticed in her as you approached her clitoris, and how she was already getting off before you went to the source, but that she froze as soon as you put your finger on her most sensitive spot. Reassure her that this is nothing to worry about. It has to do with performance anxiety. Before you touched her clitoris you were both just fooling around, both enjoying yourselves. Then when you put your finger on her spot, she felt pressure to take things higher. Go back to being more playful, and start touching her again for your own pleasure.

➣ One Stroke at a Time ⇐

Now may be a great time to introduce the idea of instant orgasm to your partner. Hopefully your partner is aware of this possibility and of the reading you've done on the subject. If necessary, describe what you've learned so far, and try to do so in a way that won't place increased pressure on your partner to perform. Let her (or him) know that you will be touching her body using a single stroke at a time. Because she was able to feel sensation in her genitals even before you touched her clitoris, you know that she can be instantly orgasmic. All she has to do, when her clitoris is touched, is focus her attention on the pleasurable feelings there.

Continue to be playful. Maybe hold a dab of lubricant directly above her clitoris without touching it, and ask her to feel. When you finally touch her clitoris, you can choose any kind of stroke that appeals to you. It can be a quick touch directly on the spot, or a long stroke upward from her perineum over her introitus and finally onto her clitoris—or any other touch you want to perform. Tell her in advance what you are doing, report any pleasure you notice, and ask her to do the same.

This whole session can be dedicated to touching her one stroke at a time. We have sometimes asked students to use *only* one single stroke, end the session, and then to write about the session. You could also graduate to some additional stroking if she has responded well to the one-stroke training—or just because both of you desire it.

➣ Graduating to More Strokes ⇐

One way to advance is to choose a specific number of strokes; for example, two or three or five. You can inform her that you will deliver, say, five direct strokes on her clitoris, then do so. Stop stroking afterward, and talk about it with her. Then you can repeat this maneuver by stroking again five times, stopping for a couple of seconds, and then stroking five more times.

Notice if she is experiencing more feeling—that is, if the sensation is increasing or decreasing. If it is increasing, you can increase the number of strokes, for example, stroking seven or ten times in a row before taking a short break. Be playful and keep communicating what you are doing. In this way she won't be surprised when you stop stroking. Keep the strokes short, stay on her favorite spot, and do not vary the kind of stroke used.

After a while, as long as she is still feeling all the strokes, you can give her a longer peak by delivering even more strokes and using your intention to keep her going. You may or may not choose to do this the first time out; remember, it is best to leave her wanting more, but do not leave her starving. Pay attention to what is going on with both of you. You want to stay in control without trying to force her to get off by continuing to touch her if she is in resistance mode. Already you've gotten her to lighten up, let go of performance anxiety, and feel far more than she's probably used to feeling.

This technique of giving just a few strokes, taking a break, and then repeating the cycle is useful for a woman who is new to this kind of attention. She is unaccustomed to having so much attention focused on her, so when you stroke her even once or twice and then stop, she will be able to get into the experience better than if you stroked her continuously. It's kind of like training with weights; you start with a small amount and gradually add more as you get stronger. Here you are adding more strokes (more stimulation) as her ability to receive attentive pleasure grows. Building one's capacity for pleasure is a shorter process than building strong muscles. Often it takes just one session to go from being able to fully feel just a couple of strokes to enjoying many. It is all about having fun; there is no specific timetable that must be met. By keeping your attention focused on the pleasure rather than the outcome, there will be less chance of creating performance anxiety. In Chapter 6 we will describe in further detail how to pleasure an untrained woman.

⇒ The Importance of Confidence ⇐

Any stimulation of a woman's genitals will be better with confidence behind it. Most women are receptive to a man who shows that he wants to learn how to give her more pleasure. They are willing to cut him some slack even when his confidence is in the budding stage. He requires practice to gain confidence, so by rewarding him for his positive attempts she will create a confident lover.

Any recipient of pleasure, whether they are a man or a woman, is more receptive to a touch that is deliberate as opposed to tentative. This is because it is much easier to surrender to someone who is self-assured than someone who is insecure about their skills. When the pleasure giver is hesitant, unsure, or timid with his or her touches, the recipient will respond negatively.

A woman can usually tell just by looking at and talking with a man how confident he really is. Self-assuredness in a potential lover makes it easier for a woman to say yes to his offers. On the flip side, some women may be put off by what they perceive as too much confidence, often described as being "cocky" or "too smooth." They may think the guy won't measure up to what he seems to promise. The key is to pay attention to the vibes she is giving off and respond accordingly. If a man notices that a woman seems afraid of his talents, he can overcome her resistances by having fun with just that notion. He can play push/pull with her, pushing her away a bit farther than she seemed prepared to go, and then reeling her back in. He can push her away by saying something like she is right to be afraid because he has been known as the "Big Bad Wolf" and he might blow her house down. Then he can say he was kidding—he is really a sheep in wolf's clothing and he will be very gentle with her and only go as far as she wants. This may be a silly little example, but you get the idea. The point is that wherever there is resistance, there is also a fun game that can be played. But the man has to enjoy playing this way. Our book *To Bed or Not to Bed* spends considerable time discussing the playful games involved in seducing someone.

⇒ Noticing and Appreciating Her ⇐

A woman who is willing to surrender and who has faith that her lover is confident and knowledgeable can be orgasmic before her partner even touches her. Just the thought of the upcoming event can be so titillating that she will be wet and turned on. All her partner has to do is to keep her on track, say some nice things, and notice and report.

Before touching your partner, take some time to gaze at her body and tell her how beautiful she is. Detail what you find so attractive—her eyes or her thighs or her skin or whatever. It's important to be honest, of course. Most women love to be noticed and flattered, and doing so will help her know that you are truly enjoying what you are doing. You can also tell her that she has a "beautiful pussy" and a "gorgeous clitoris." Pay attention to her face and notice if she is appreciating your flattery or if it is too much for her to handle. Unless a person is good at hiding their feelings, observing their face can easily tell you what emotion they're experiencing. Notice when you speak to them whether you are taking them higher or lower emotionally. Only continue with a particular line of communication if they enjoy it.

You can tell when a person is ready to be touched—wants physical contact —and when they are afraid or reluctant. As long as you sense any resistance in your partner, proceed cautiously; even take a step back if necessary. You can say something like, "We don't have to do this, but if we do, it is going to be a hell of a lot of fun." Once in bed, a woman still has to be continually seduced. By this we mean that you always want her coming toward you, desiring more pleasure, and if she is not, then you have to tease her by threatening to stop.

➤ Time to Touch ◄

When you can no longer resist touching her, then it must be time to do so. Avoid diving for the clitoris; rather, approach it slowly and deliberately, using any of the techniques we've described so far. Start from wherever you feel inclined to touch her. Remember that a light stroke is more exciting than a firm one.

I enjoy letting my hands go almost on autopilot; that is, touching without too much thinking or planning. (I still remain aware of all of my partner's responses, however.) Just go with the flow, allowing your hands to touch wherever they feel like it. Training and practice help you develop an instinct for how to touch. As with any skill, once you learn the proper techniques you become freed up to go outside the box, so to speak. I may use the back of my hands, my wrist, or even my whole forearm. Of course, my fingers and palms have to get in on the act. Always remember to touch for your own pleasure. There is no map; each time out will be different and special.

Report any signs of pleasure that you notice, and compliment her on anything that you find attractive and appealing. If you find a special curve that is sexy or gorgeous, do not keep it to yourself; inform her immediately. If you like the way she feels, or the softness of her pubic hair, let her know. If you enjoy her scent, describe how she has a wonderfully perfumed fragrance that is delicious to inhale. Women can be quite sensitive about the way their pussies smell, so if you compliment her aroma she will feel more like surrendering to her pleasure.

Remember that your confidence, your enjoyment, your sweet talk, your playfulness, and of course your attention and intention all have an effect on how willing she is to surrender. The more she is willing to surrender, the more she will be able to feel, and the more instantaneously orgasmic she will be. You want to cause her to be willing to let go and lower her defenses, putting all her energy into experiencing sensation, *sensation*, **sensation.** If she does this, she will be in orgasm before you even get to her clitoris.

If she lets loose and goes for the sensation, keep doing what you're doing. With more of the same kind of attention from you, as long as she continues to be receptive, you can take her higher and higher.

Handling Resistances: Enemies of Turn-On

If, on the other hand, you encounter resistance, you have a number of choices. You can proceed with caution and give her some delicious strokes and see if there is anyone home, or you can let her know that you sense resistance and ask her some questions. The questions can range from asking her if she really wants pleasure now, to asking her what she is thinking about. She may be afraid that she won't feel as much as she "should," or that somehow she will fail in your eyes. Allay her doubts by letting her know that you are doing this for your own fun and pleasure. Remind her that by placing her attention on these negative ideas she is resisting her own pleasure, and that it is time for her to invest in her pleasure by focusing on fun and sexy thoughts. Increasing the communication is usually your best chance at overcoming the resistance and getting her to a place of greater surrender. Look at her face when you ask the questions and you will see if you are making any headway or if your audience has checked out.

We often tell people that the two biggest enemies of turn-on are doubt and anger. We've spent a lot of time in our earlier books discussing these topics, and we want to repeat here that as long as a person is feeling angry or having doubts they cannot place their attention on pleasurable sensation. You cannot have attention on your anger and on your pleasure at the same time. You have to choose. You must doubt your doubt and deliberately focus your attention on your pleasure.

Doubt will keep a person, especially a woman, from letting go and allowing herself to feel as intensely as she can. The doubt can be about almost anything—how she looks, whether her clitoris is big enough, whether her labia are too big, how her genitals smell, whether this is the right thing to do, whether he is just planning to stick it in later.

If you decide to deal with the resistance by continuing stroking, it is still in everyone's best interest to keep the communication open. Let her know that you are not feeling much response coming from her and that you are going to continue because you want to see what happens if you keep touching her. Sometimes people just require a little bit of time and a little more stimulation before they can focus their attention on what is occurring in their body. As long as you are open about the fact that you don't sense much pleasurable energy emanating from her body, at least she can trust that you are telling her the truth. Make sure she is not tensing up and waiting to feel something in the future.

If she argues with you by claiming that she feels more than you think she does, again it would be best to stop and determine exactly what is going on. Likewise, if you do continue and observe no increase in sensual energy, it is time to stop and take a longer break.

⇒ Integrity ⇐

In response to her resistance, let's say you have asked her some questions and she has answered honestly. It is okay to start touching her again whenever it feels right to do so. But know that you must trust your own feelings and have the integrity to follow through with how you really feel. Most men are production junkies; that is, they want to give their partners pleasure no matter what. That may be a great attitude for succeeding in business or warfare, but it is not the best attitude to embrace when producing pleasure. A man has to realize that proceeding full steam ahead, damn the torpedoes, will not work in this scenario. Creating sensual pleasure is more like practicing certain martial arts, where one uses the opponent's resistance to throw them. So the best move may be to back off and somehow make her come toward you. You could say something like, "I'd love to give you more, but it just does not seem that you want more" or, "I was having such a lovely time with you up till now, but it seems that you've had enough. Am I mistaken?"

A student was in our program to learn how to have bigger and better orgasms. We had a couple of sessions a day with her, and the morning sessions were consistently more intense than the afternoon sessions. One day, just before the scheduled afternoon session, we mentioned this to her, said we wondered if she might be tired by the afternoon, and suggested taking a break from the second session that day. She agreed with us about her progress (which is a good sign), and said yes she was tired and felt we were right to suggest not proceeding to the bedroom that afternoon. As soon as she agreed with us and realized she did not have to engage in any sensual activity, she opened up and turned on. We picked this up and told her that whereas she seemed flat before, we were now feeling quite a bit of desire coming from her. We told her we could change directions and have some fun, as now it seemed she was open to it. We quickly went to the bedroom and had our best session yet. By reading a person properly, telling them what we see, and having them agree with us, we can free up of a lot of energy that can be used for having fun.

⤜ Getting into Agreement ⤛

It is really important that the person receiving the pleasure agree with the analysis of the person producing the pleasure. When we call a person on some behavior, the moment they agree with our viewpoint they release some form of resistance. The agreement seems to allow the flow of energy to increase. Things will only get better from there. It is a form of surrender to say, "Yes, you are right; you hit the nail on the head." As a man and often the pleasure giver, I really appreciate it when this happens. If my partner were to deny my feelings and argue with me, it would just create more resistance. Even if the other person is sure of their case, arguing about it does not bode well for their pleasure.

This, of course, does not mean that they cannot ask for something they want or correct an uncomfortable touch they are receiving. We just encourage them to do so in a way that is also pleasurable; for example, using the three-step training cycle. In other words, it helps to move things along smoothly if you can first get into agreement with the pleasure giver and only then bring up what you would like to change. There are many books on the market that discuss good communication techniques and how to promote interpersonal harmony, even when you think you disagree with the other person. One such book is *Peace in Everyday Relationships,* by Sheila Alson and Gayle B. Burnett. If you believe you could benefit from this sort of training, we encourage you to pursue it further.

What we are actually describing here is the best way to respond to someone else's viewpoints that are focused on your pleasure. Do you want to be right or do you want to have pleasure? Do you want your anger or do you want your pleasure?

The woman in the above example was not even in bed yet when she decided to be agreeable. This scenario clearly demonstrates the power of saying yes and surrendering and being in agreement with the way things are. It illustrates how the orgasm often begins long before the actual going to bed and the tangible touching start. The dance begins when two people are just beginning to plan and talk about the pleasure that is available.

⤜ A Tangent? ⤛

Here we are in the middle of a description of how to pleasure a partner, and we keep getting closer to describing the techniques and then going off on some tangent about seducing your partner's mind. This is not an accident. The most important part of giving someone pleasure is focusing your attention on them, and the most important part of pleasuring a woman is getting into her mind. If you are unable to seduce a woman's mind, she is not going to surrender her body. Our pattern of repeatedly moving in and backing off, then, is no tangent but an actual seductive technique that anyone who wishes to become a master at giving pleasure needs to know. The attention-focusing techniques that are so important to the seduction will also prove vital when touching for pleasure.

⮞ Reasserting Control ⮜

Some people avoid pleasure in bed by bringing up a topic related to everyday business. Your response depends on what kind of a distraction it presents. If it is brief and fun you can play with it by saying something like, "Oh, you would rather talk about that than about your pleasure."

Sometimes the pleasure recipient will start to touch or stroke the body of the pleasure giver. This can be okay if agreed upon by both parties in advance. The important matter is whether the action serves to distract the recipient from focusing on her or his pleasure. Often it is a test to see if they can lessen your degree of control.

In response to any of these scenarios, keep things playful. Use your seductive wiles with even more intent. Use push/pull till you get your partner out of the position of delegating the action. The fastest way to regain control is to get into agreement, so do not argue with them, and by all means do not just keep on rubbing on them. Instead, agree that it is time to do something different, that they probably have had enough stimulation. Push them further than they expect you to. Then you will be back in the driver's seat and can suggest new ideas.

⮞ The Role of Chemistry ⮜

What almost every recipient of pleasure wants is to find someone with whom they feel safe enough to give it up to. Lust, or chemistry, usually counts, too. They really do not want to win by taking over the controlling position. They may want to test you, however, to make sure you are a good partner for them to surrender to.

Some married couples may encounter problems concerning surrendering—mostly because they have misplaced part of the lust they originally had for each other. Some married people, often women, have allowed repressed anger to build up for years, and you know what that does to turn-on. Deliberately seeking to enhance the pleasure in their marriage can help a couple move beyond even old anger. Still, sometimes getting help from a professional therapist is necessary. One way to keep the pleasure-to-anger ratio high in a relationship is to keep your communications up-to-date. Avoid letting any negative feelings fester; make sure you express them as soon as you can. It may sound like a cliché, but communication is vitally important if you want to continue growing as a couple.

Remember, too, that even in long-term partnerships, a woman can always decide to turn up her "lust button," which means she can touch her partner in such a way that he will have no choice but to surrender. She doesn't have to look like a supermodel to work this charm. She has to be in love with herself, enjoy herself, and take pleasure in what she is doing. She has to focus attention on her partner, noticing the things that turn him on, such as exposing some skin or touching him on his favorite spot or whatever. And, of course, by adding some sexy talk into the mix she can up the lust scale. Saying things that are sensual or nasty is a good idea for both women and men who want to reintroduce some lust and fun into their sexual activities. Knowing your partner's fantasies can be helpful in determining what to say and what not to say to make them yearn to be touched by you. Seduction is really a mental game, and like any game the more you play the better you become.

Men do not have a lust button to call with, but they do have their wits and their seductive capabilities. To turn on a woman, a man must give her reasons to feel more intensely. Ways of doing this include talking and paying her lots of attention. Noticing and complimenting her before you get into the bedroom are excellent starting places. If you wait till you get her into the bedroom, it may be too difficult. More likely, she will resist even going that far. Another seduction technique for men is to learn the ways of pleasuring women; hopefully you are doing this if you have read this far.

When partners first get together there are usually lots of chemical and hormonal catalysts available to spark the pleasure. But many couples who at first used chemistry to ignite their love lives are no longer having much fun in the bedroom. After a number of years the chemistry transforms from physical abandon and attraction to love and caring. Sometimes the chemistry fades if there haven't been any positive emotional additions to the relationship. Furthermore, most people have not learned or trained themselves or their partners about pleasuring, specifically about how to give a woman pleasure. Couples who come to us to learn how to use their hands to give each other pleasure greatly enhance the quality of their sex lives. The addition of these skills can increase the level of fun in the bedroom far more than chemistry alone and can lead to a lifetime full of intimate encounters.

⋙ Hand Placement (on a Woman's Body) ⋘

So now you're touching your partner, wanting to provide her with instantly orgasmic sensations. How should you position your hands for maximum effect? I'm right-handed, so I usually like to place my left hand so that it's holding onto the woman's buttocks with the thumb at the base of her introitus (see Figure 8). This allows for lots of contact and gives her a sense of relaxing into my hand. I do not insert my thumb inside her vagina unless it is invited—that is, more or less sucked in. The placement of thumb at the introitus allows me to easily gauge the strength of her orgasmic contractions. Remember, now that you're touching erectile tissue, use lots of lubricant.

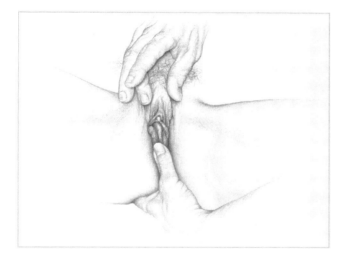

Figure 8.
Placement of second hand, thumb at base of introitus

We once had a student who'd recently had some medical problems. Because of these issues she did not want anyone putting a finger inside her vagina, let alone a penis, as she felt that any sort of insertion caused her irritation. She did not want me using my hand on her in the way described above (with my thumb at the base of her introitus), so we tried a number of different positions to overcome this resistance while also incorporating some method for me to gauge the strength of her contractions. The solution we came up with was for me to press the knuckles of my left fist gently against her perineum to monitor the contractions. At other times I gently placed one left finger a little higher into the introitus, closer to the clitoris (see Figure 9). Sometimes, at the beginning of a session, I used only my right hand to stroke her and did not use my left hand at all. Usually, after a few minutes of my stimulating her clitoris, she would relax enough to let me put my thumb and left hand in the formation we'd agreed upon.

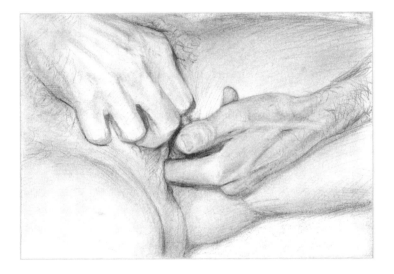

Figure 9. *Finger of second hand placed gently at introitus*

⋟ More Signs of Resistance ⋞

The above scenario is an example of how to deal with a partner's resistance. If I had tried to convince this student that she had to submit to my expertise, she would have built up greater resistance and we would have gotten nowhere. A willingness on Vera's and my part to change direction and adapt to the special circumstances—while remaining playful about it—allowed us to overcome her resistance. Later in her training she permitted me to position my hands any way that I wanted, including resting my thumb at the base of her introitus. She knew she could trust me not to do anything she didn't want, and this opened her up to surrendering to her pleasure.

As you've seen throughout this chapter, resistance to receiving pleasure can show up in many different forms. The expert giver of pleasure will be able to spot any of these quickly and do what is necessary to move the focus back to feeling and enjoying orgasmic pleasure. We will wrap this chapter up by listing a few more common signs of resistance and discussing how to counteract them.

Too Many Requests for Change

Sometimes the person receiving pleasure will want to change too many variables all at once—the music, the lighting, the position, and so on—which may cause you to sense that you are losing control as the pleasure giver. Tell your partner that you appreciate their input and that you will decide which of their ideas can be assimilated. You must determine where to draw the line. Otherwise they will keep pushing the envelope, and you will no longer be creating pleasure for them.

Excessive Appreciation

Occasionally a person will do too much talking, saying over and over how great it is and how much fun they are having. If what your partner is saying does not jibe with the way you are sensing the experience, speak up and let your partner know how you feel. Pretending to be in ecstasy does not make it so. It is merely one more way to distract oneself from feeling and approving of what actually is happening. Tell your partner that you like it when they verbally acknowledge their pleasure, but you only want them to do so when they are really feeling it. They do not have to prove how much they are feeling, because you are there too and can tell when they are overdoing it. The goal of approving is to help them feel more, and if they are trying to convince you how much pleasure they are having, they will have little attention left for feeling. Yes, it is great to verbalize one's appreciation, and when it is done in response to how much pleasure one is really feeling, it comes out easily and everyone enjoys hearing it. Just don't overdo it.

Similarly, when a person moans and makes noises, the sounds emanating from them hopefully add to the pleasure of everyone involved. Sometimes people will fake pleasure by making more noise than seems appropriate. If this happens, you are advised to point this discrepancy out. When the sounds interfere with the pleasure, the person will benefit by being told to knock it off (in a nice way, of course). We had a student whose sounds simply did not equate with the poor way she was getting off. She may have fooled others in the past who were not as experienced as we are, but when we pointed out that her moans did not match up with her orgasmic abilities she quickly agreed that she was faking it and appreciated that somebody had noticed.

Shaking

When a person reaches a point of ecstasy that is higher than they've ever felt before, their leg may start to shake. At this point you can ask them to relax, or to do "push outs," which can stop their body from tensing up. A push out is an action of the PC (pubococcygeal) muscle, which surrounds the genital and anal area in the shape of a figure eight. To push it out, you deliberately push the muscle downward as though you were urinating. Push out for a few seconds, then relax the muscle. Keep breathing normally the whole time. To help train a student to do push outs, we may insert a finger into her vagina and ask her to push the finger out. You do not have to put your finger in too deeply, it just has to be deep enough so that a person can push it out.

If the leg continues to shake, depending on how intense the shaking is, we may keep stimulating the genitals or we may stop altogether. If the shaking seems minor and seems not to interfere with the pleasure, it is okay to continue with the stimulation as long as the pleasure keeps rising.

Fast Breathing

Some responders start to breathe fast when the sensation gets stronger than what they are used to. Again, ask them to relax and breathe as regularly as they can. Slightly faster breathing is a normal bodily response to orgasm, but when it becomes a distraction it is no longer a normal response.

The Too-Sensitive Clitoris

We touched on the topic of extreme clitoral sensitivity in Chapter 2. We have encountered this scenario quite often and have received numerous e-mails about it. An extremely sensitive clitoris actually presents the woman with an opportunity to start coming before her clitoris is even touched. Utilize all of the information we've included about feeling your partner's hand as it hovers above the clitoris. Women who are supersensitive should be able to feel changes in air pressure as their partner moves a hand or a finger in the air directly over the clitoris.

Some women can appreciate this indirect stimulation, but others are actually quite turned off to any pleasure and will resist any kind of direct or indirect sensation. Some women simply have never been touched directly on the clitoris and are afraid. But in other cases extreme resistance indicates psychological issues emanating from molestation or abuse that occurred in the past. Sometimes these issues can be cleared up with lots of kind attention from a partner who is willing to talk about their secret, and other times the person will need to receive psychological help. We are not therapists, so we do not claim to be able to help those who require this kind of assistance. For less traumatized individuals, start with a lot of talking. Encourage them to forgive themselves for whatever happened in the past. They can learn to leave those incidents in the past and stop carrying them around in the present, or at least stop allowing them to consciously affect their behavior.

Whenever we have worked with a woman who has claimed to be too sensitive to be touched, we have found that by paying slow, deliberate attention to her fears and desires we were able to overcome this obstacle and get her to the place where she enjoyed being touched directly on her clitoris. Take as much time as is necessary to move past this fear. There is no rush, and if you demonstrate this to someone who has this fear it will help her become more trusting and willing to explore new possibilities.

Certainly do not go in with guns blasting and think you will conquer her that way. Have fun with the situation by enjoying her sensitivity. You can touch her all over her body, gradually moving closer to her genitals. Lightly graze over her pubic hair with the back of your hand. When you finally get to her genitals you can check out the sensitivity of her perineum, her introitus, and her labia, but do not touch her clitoris.

Now pleasurably spread some lubricant all over her genitals (except, of course, her clitoris). See the section in the next chapter where we describe in detail how to apply lubricant. Employing a delicate pressure, you can stimulate her labia using one stroke at a time or a series of strokes. Keep lightly stroking all over her genitals, except you know where. You can place your finger above her clitoris without touching and ask if this creates too much pressure. You can pull back her hood with your other hand and again place your finger above the exposed clitoris, still not touching it, and ask if she would like more pressure. You can stop at any point or even go back to stroking her labia.

If she does ask for more pressure, apply a large glob of lubricant to your fingertip. Still pulling back the hood, slowly and deliberately make your way toward the clitoris, letting her know how close you are getting. Now gently touch the clitoris with the dab of lubricant that is on your finger. (This is a case when using a more viscous lubricant, such as one containing petroleum jelly, works better than using a lubricant with a thin, liquid consistency.) Remove your finger, and ask if she would like more stimulation. She probably will, and in that case you can touch your lubricant-laden finger to her clitoris and give her one stroke. Ask if she would like another. You are on your way, and if you continue in this slow and deliberate manner she soon will be eating out of your hand.

$\sim$

In the next chapter we will continue by describing specific strokes and presenting additional ideas for pleasuring.

CHAPTER 5

A Variety
of Pleasurable Touches

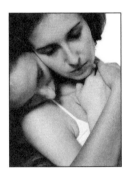

*T*his chapter discusses different types of touch that can be added to your bag of tricks for pleasuring your partner. Most of these are preliminary strokes to tease your partner or trigger sensation before you get to the most sensitive spots on your partner's clitoris or penis. Still, these touches can be extremely pleasurable in themselves and can demonstrate once again how a single touch can cause orgasmic feelings. We go into detail about how to sensually spread lubricant on your lover's genitals. At the end of the chapter we introduce a specific clitoral stroke.

⇒ Pulling, Stretching, and Applying Pressure ⇐

One of the things I enjoy doing, and that many women seem to enjoy having done to them, is to pull or stretch the skin around the clitoris without directly touching the clitoris. You'll want to get a good view of the genitals before doing any deliberate stroking. Place your hands on both sides of her outer labia and pull them apart (see Figure 2 on page 34). Most women seem to enjoy the sensation and the attention of this action. It is the gentlemanly thing to do at this point to comment on how pretty or sexy or beautiful her pussy is. She is very exposed, and a nice comment from you will help her surrender to what you are doing. Some women will be instantly orgasmic even with just this small amount of preliminary attention. If you notice any contractions, or other signs of orgasm such as wetness or engorgement, let her know, as this adds to her sensation. Maintain some pressure on the labia by stretching them outward for as long as both partners are enjoying it. You can incrementally add more pressure to find out what feels best to your partner.

When you are first learning about your partner's genitals, adequate lighting is vital. Most people are conditioned to doing "it" in the dark, under the covers. We are not asking you to give this up but rather to add to your repertoire some new ways of having pleasure, including with the lights on and on top of the covers.

Most guys also appreciate it when a woman takes time to focus some admiring attention on their genitals, although this seems to be somewhat less important to men. Before a woman lubricates and starts stroking the penis, or before she puts it into her mouth and starts licking and sucking, it feels good to have her move the pubic hair out of the way and execute some pressing or stretching or pulling movements.

Here's a fun motion that both men and women enjoy. Place your palm firmly over the pubic area, above the genitals, and tug upward. Start with light pressure and incrementally add more while asking your partner if they would like increased pressure. (We discuss this touch in detail below.) Once you know your partner's preferences you can immediately use their favorite pressure if you wish. People's preferences do change over time, so it is a good idea to check in with your partner once in a while.

⇒ Exposing Her Clitoris ⇐

The upward tugging described in the previous section will generally expose a woman's clitoris from under the hood (see Figure 3 on page 35). Remark how beautiful and sexy her clitoris is. You can ask her to feel the air on it or even blow a puff of air onto it with your mouth. You will be surprised at how much pressure most women can enjoy on their mons area. The more pressure you are able to exert here, the more exposed her clitoris becomes. Being able to expose the clitoris is very important, because as long as the clitoris is hiding under the hood, you will be unable to take complete control and reach the full potential of her sensations. Exposing it properly will facilitate access to all areas of the clitoris and make your job much easier than if you were digging in the dark. Some women enjoy this move so much that strong visible contractions may result each time you tug.

Another playful way to expose her clitoris is to position two or three fingers above the hood and pull back (see Figure 4 on page 35). To increase her pleasure, you can press your fingers into her body. Again, learn exactly how she likes it by starting lightly and incrementally progressing to greater levels of pressure.

For another technique she may really enjoy, place your index finger on one side of her clitoral hood and your middle finger on the other side, pads down, and, while applying pressure upward and inward, pull back on the hood to expose the clitoris. You can play with squeezing the hood and clitoris together between your two fingers, varying the amount of pressure applied. As always, begin with a small amount of pressure and continuously ask if she would like more. Once you learn what her preferences are, you can be more playful and perhaps somewhat less inquisitive.

Sometimes I like to put the tip of one finger against the clitoral hood and exert pressure toward the clitoris (see Figure 10 on the next page), which allows me to touch the different quadrants of the clitoris through the hood. I am not really stroking, just pushing inward. Nor am I exposing the clitoris here, but deliberately giving her pleasure through the hood. Some women will show signs of orgasm with this touch; again, report any such signs that you notice. Be sure to communicate with her in advance about what you are doing, keep her informed during your touching, and ask questions that she can easily answer about her preferences for more or less pressure.

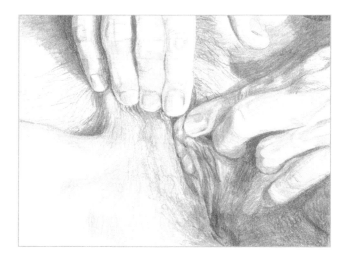

Figure 10. *Pressing the clitoris indirectly through the hood*

Try placing your index finger and thumb on either side of the clitoral hood (see Figure 11). Now gently squeeze and release, squeeze and release, using incrementally increasing pressure. You will be surprised at how much pressure you will be able to exert. A fun little stroke to use from this position is to

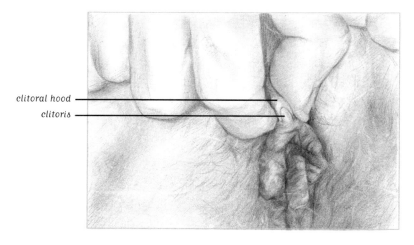

clitoral hood ——

clitoris ——

Figure 11. *Putting pressure on both sides of clitoral hood*

squeeze the hood in a kind of rocking motion so that the clitoris moves in and out and up and down. We call this one the Yo-Yo stroke. With it, you can practice instant orgasm one slow squeeze at a time, with a long pause between squeezes, or you can go faster, making the clitoris bounce up and down.

Later in the chapter we describe more ways to expose the clitoris (see the section "Retract the Hood").

➤ Pressure on the Lower Abdomen ◄

We've briefly described how to press with your palm either above the pubic hair on the lower abdomen, or slightly farther down, directly on the pubic bone. Not everyone will like this move but many people do, both men and women. Your partner may enjoy this more after she or he has been stroked for a while on the clitoris or penis and is already in orgasm or feeling intense sensations. I really like to have this area pressed down and released while a woman is stroking my penis (see Figure 5 on page 37).

In conjunction with your strokes on your partner's genitals, you can press down and release, press down and release. No lubricant is necessary in this location as it is not erectile tissue and you are not really rubbing but rather pressing and stretching. Try pressing and stretching in all the different directions to determine which directions, how much pressure, and which speeds feel best to you and your partner. Some people may feel orgasmic just from doing this, so keep an open mind and enjoy the play. You can also press and stretch the lower abdominal or pubic area as you simultaneously press through the hood to the clitoris with the fingers of your other hand.

➤ Pressure on Her Entire Vulva ◄

Put your hand over her entire genital area, with the heel of your hand on the pubic bone and your fingers pointed downward. From here you can use your fingers to press against the perineum or lower labia or buttocks cheeks, and use your palm to press against the upper labia and the clitoral area. Alternate applying pressure first to one area and then to another. Notice any signs of orgasm, such as contractions or wetness. Tell your partner what you are sensing and how much you're enjoying yourself.

You can also use this touch while lying next to your partner without look-ing at her genitals (see Figure 12). It's not necessary here to be too precise in your movements; just have fun and feel the pleasure, which are always the goals. Sometimes using very little motion—for example, by just placing your hand on her genital area and leaving it there—produces much pleasure. Of course, avoid leaving your hand stationary for too long. As we have explained, the way to maximize sensation is to create differences in sensation. If you keep your hand in one position or use a particular stroke for too long, your part-ner's positive feelings will eventually fade. After keeping your hand still for a while, add a little squeezing and releasing. This can be a fun way for your part-ner to practice feeling the burst of attention that triggers instant orgasm. Ask your partner to refocus her attention with each cycle of squeeze/release.

Figure 12.
Lying side-by-side
with a partner

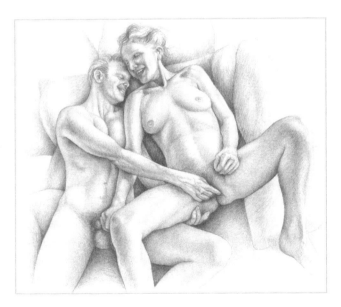

Sometimes, before any stroking, I will press my fist against a woman's perineum and introitus area. I may use my other hand to pull her clitoral hood upward (see Figure 13). From here I can alternate where I apply pressure, no-tice her response, and report what I see. Again, some women, especially those who have a highly developed capacity for orgasm, will feel great pleasure with this move and even show signs of orgasm.

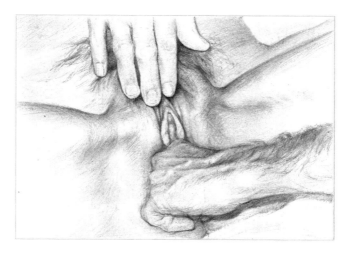

Figure 13. *Pressure on perineum and mons*

⇒ Squeezing His Penis ⇐

Women, you can create a lot of pleasure in your man by squeezing his penis, even without progressing to any other types of touches. Of course, this could also be a way to merely start the action. Press with your fist against his perineum (see Figure 14). Take delight in touching and holding the penis, the scrotum, and the whole genital area, from the lower abdomen to the anus.

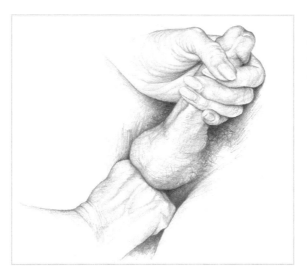

Figure 14.
Applying pressure to his perineum while squeezing his penis

You can begin by touching his penis through his clothes, which can feel great if you take pleasure in doing so. You do not have to use much motion—sometimes the less activity the better. I have leaked semen on more than one occasion from sensing a woman's desire without her even having touched my penis. When she does touch me the feeling can increase, but if she didn't want to touch me yet and did so anyway, the feeling can subside. You can put your hand down your guy's pants or open his zipper. You can undo his belt and pull down his pants, or request that he do so. Guaranteed he will enjoy the attention.

You can also try just holding the naked penis in your hand, without using any motion. Play with different amounts of pressure by lightly squeezing the penis with your full hand, and then incrementally adding more pressure till both parties find their favorite levels of pressure. Once you know what level of pressure he prefers, you can squeeze for a few seconds and then stop. In this way you can get him to feel more intensely using just one stroke or one squeeze, while communicating what you are doing so he will not be left wondering. Repeat this sequence one squeeze at a time, as long as both you and he stay interested. Try pulling at the same time that you are squeezing. Of course you'll need to find out how much pulling he prefers before it hurts. Experiment to see how much squeezing goes best with how much pulling. You can have a wonderful time doing this research.

Take his scrotum, or his balls, in your hand. Just put your hand around the balls and feel them. If you do it with hands pointing down, your finger pads can either curl up behind the scrotum or can touch his perineum area. At first simply hold the scrotum in your hand without applying too much pressure—just enough so that you do not appear tentative or hesitant. They are yours to play with; all you have to do is keep the communication lines open. Just hold and feel and report anything to your partner that you notice. You can place your wrist over his penis so that you can touch his whole genital area with one hand. You may notice some engorgement or some movement of the testicles. Keep letting your partner know what you are sensing.

At some point you can play with applying varying amounts of pressure to his perineum. You can pull on the scrotum, again starting with light pressure and incrementally adding more, after asking him if he would like more. Most men enjoy having their scrotum played with, and as long as you avoid pushing the testes into the body you can experiment, using lots of communication to find out what feels best. Press your fingers against his "hidden penis" (the engorged area that you can feel through his perineum), his prostate area, or any other place that you wish to touch.

Get creative. You can wrap your hand around his penis and pull. Of course you should ask him if he would like more pulling, and increase in small increments until you know exactly how he likes it. He may prefer different amounts of pressure on different days, so it is always a good idea to ask if you aren't sure. At the same time, it is also important to touch him as though you own his genitals. You can place one or both hands anywhere down there, positioning them in any way that feels good to you. Tug his scrotum downward while pulling his penis in the opposite direction. A fun little exercise is to hold his penis for him while he urinates, just to see what it feels like. The object here isn't to turn him on too much, only to gain more knowledge about his penis.

➣ More Ways to Touch a Woman ➢

We've talked about the importance of starting your sensual play with a woman by touching her genitals in areas other than the clitoris itself. First do so without lubricant and with light stroking, maybe using the back of your hand or wrist, tickling her pubic hair. Then add some lubricant and touch very lightly, avoiding getting too much lube in the pubic hair. Be playful and touch her in any way you want, as long as she remains responsive. Use your forearm, fist, or elbow, with or without lubricant. Touch around the lips, and press your arm, hand, or elbow against her entire vulva. Include the clitoral area or not, depending on how you feel. When a person is very excited, touching them in this way can bring them down a bit, back into their bodies, so to speak. You can press and release, repeating as many times as it is appreciated. One of our students, when first experimenting with our EMO techniques, liked having an elbow pressed against her vulva more than she liked direct clitoral stimulation. When you are being playful with your partner and doing things like touching her with an elbow or forearm, she can relax and feel less intimidated, which will allow her to receive heightened sensation.

Take your time. Move close to the clitoris and then back away. Ask if she can feel your finger hovering above her clitoris. Repeat this as long as it is fun for the both of you. Women can play with a guy's penis in this way, too, getting close to it without touching it and communicating to him while doing so. This is a good way for the pleasure recipient to learn how to place more attention on her or his genitals. It is the path to instant orgasm.

To build trust, you can spend an entire session enjoying this delicate, slow dance, getting close without quite getting there. If you sense that she would appreciate a little touch on the clitoris, let her know that you are going to pull back her hood and touch her lightly with a little bit of lubricant for just one stroke. See how that goes; if direct contact goes well then do it again. If it is too much, then back off and return to stroking the labia or elsewhere. Sometimes I will hold my finger very close to her clitoris and ask her to reach for my finger. We do not want her to move her body, and we let her know this in advance, but the clitoris can engorge and at times will actually come toward my finger.

➢ Lubrication ➢

Lubricating someone's genitals can trigger lots of pleasure, even orgasmic sensations. You can tease your partner by saying that applying lubricant may be all you do today. I usually like to start at the perineum and work my way slowly toward the clitoris, without actually applying any lube directly onto the clitoris until after the whole genital area is lubricated and I am ready to stroke it.

It is very important to apply the lubricant in a sensual fashion. I know for myself that a good application of lubricant makes a huge difference in how well I am able to surrender to the person hoping to pleasure me. When there is no special tenderness or attention being focused on me as my partner applies lubricant, it does not bode well for the rest of the session. However, when a woman applies lubricant with finesse and caring gentleness and takes pleasure in doing it, I can completely surrender myself into her hands and let go of all my resistances. The same is true when applying lubricant to a woman's genitals. The more confident and attentive you are, and the more you enjoy the act, the easier it will be for her to relax and surrender to what you *are* doing and what you *will be* doing to her. I also know from my own masturbation experiences that I may not feel all that turned-on before I apply lubricant to my genitals, but if I take my time and pleasurably spread the lubricant I can immediately go into a state of great anticipation. This is true if you are doing it to yourself or to someone else. Spreading lubricant is therefore one of the most important parts of the sensual cycle and is not to be taken for granted or done with incomplete attention.

Since the main goal of this book is to get you to feel more from the very first moments of the sensual encounter, you can understand how important it is to apply lubricant with as much enjoyment and attention as possible. When you're applying lubricant, encourage your partner to experience the process with as much sensitivity and abandon as they can. Do this by communicating your own enjoyment as you are spreading the lube. The act itself is so sensual that if you want your partner to get as much as possible out of it, they need to feel totally taken care of.

I usually get a large dab of lubricant from the jar and put it on the back of my second hand. This way I do not have to go back to the jar after touching my partner's genitals or anal area. As we've said, this technique works best with a more viscous, oil-based lube.

I lubricate a woman's genitals somewhat differently every time, depending on the circumstances and how I feel, even with the same person. I may stay on the perineum for a couple of minutes, stroking up and down, or I may quickly coat the area with lubricant and move on. I then start playing with her labia minora or inner lips (see Figure 1 on page 33). I will often put a little lube on the tip of my finger, and then lubricate and stimulate one side at a time. I may go from the bottom to the top of the labia, noting how smooth and wonderful it feels. Up and down, up and down, with light teasing pressure I move closer to her clitoris and retreat. I will then go to the other side and do the same kind of playful stroke. When I rub on Vera this way she is already having strong contractions and enjoying it tremendously. New students often enjoy this kind of teasing a lot, though the contractions, if any, may not be strong. It may be a good idea to ask your partner to "feel the lubricant being spread." You can even get more specific and say things like "Feel your left labia as I slowly glide up its length."

After spreading lubricant on the inner labia, I enjoy spreading some on the introitus, the opening to the vagina, which lies just inside the labia. With a bit of lubricant on my fingertip, I like to start from the base of the introitus and work my way toward the clitoris, and then slowly retreat back downward. I continue going up and down as long as it is fun for both of us. When I get close to the clitoris I often notice my partner's level of sensation rising. After the introitus is well lubed I may place my entire middle finger lengthwise along it, pads down, moving the finger slightly or applying a little pressure. At this point I may do the Michael Douglas stroke (see Figure 7 on page 62), applying pressure till I can feel the clitoral shaft against my finger. By applying slightly more pressure I can often feel the shaft engorging. By releasing and pressing again, I can often trigger a high degree of pleasurable sensation, even orgasmic contractions. As always, remember to use incrementally increasing amounts of pressure to learn her preferences.

Or I may take a small glob of lubricant and quickly lubricate her entire genital area, starting from the perineum. I almost always leave the clitoral hood and the clitoris itself dry. The reason we do this is to make the clitoris the focal point. When it is not touched or lubricated, it remains the center of attention, which creates desire in the woman to have it touched. Furthermore, you never want to lubricate the hood, because eventually you want to pull it back away from the clitoris, and lubricating it would make it too slippery. For the same reason, I don't put any lubricant on the thumb of my stroking hand—it is often used to pull back the hood. If you forget and spread lube on the clitoral hood or on the thumb of your stroking hand, just have a towel close by and dry it off.

The most important thing to remember in applying the lubricant—or in employing any sensual technique—is to have fun doing it. You can make up your own ways to lubricate, using one finger, two fingers, or even the whole hand.

Some people, both women and men, really enjoy having their anal area played with. If that is the case make sure your partner cleans up back there before entering the bedroom. Then you can apply your favorite lubricant. Again, enjoy the application, communicate about what you are going to do before doing it, and ask questions to learn your partner's preferences. You do not have to use any insertion at this point—or at any time, for that matter.

Once you have finished lubricating her genitals, you are ready to begin the stroking in earnest. You don't have to, however; you can continue to play with her genitals, still avoiding her clitoris till she is really ready to be touched there. The entire genital area is well lubricated now, so you have a whole playing field available; don't be in a rush to get to the clitoris.

➤ Lubricating a Man ➤

As I said above, I love it when a woman takes her time to sensually lubricate my penis. Before starting, it is a good idea to brush all pubic hairs, loose or attached, out of the way. If your partner is not circumcised, pull the foreskin down away from the head of the penis and remove any stray hairs from that area as well. Let him know what you are doing, and take pleasure in the process.

I like it when my partner applies a glob of lubricant directly to my penis. Other men may prefer that the lubricant first be warmed up in their partner's hands. You can start slowly on the top side of the penis with a light, up-and-down application. Then, using a little more lubricant, apply it to the underside, working your way slowly to the apex or frenulum, the corona, and the head or glans, making sure to cover every square millimeter with lubricant.

You can use light or more firm pressure; check in with your partner about his preferences, using yes-or-no questions as described in Chapter 3. You could even drip lubricant straight from the bottle onto his genitals. You can coat one or both of your hands with lubricant and slowly or quickly rub your hand(s) up and down the shaft and head. You can dab a little lubricant at a time on a small area, repeating until the entire penis is coated. You could use an edible lubricant and spread it with your lips. You could put some lubricant on your big toe and spread it with your feet. There are obviously myriad ways to play with lubricant; the bottom line, as always, is to enjoy the act. By checking out different types of lube and different strokes, a couple can learn a lot about how he likes to be pleasured, perhaps even discovering new things in the process.

➤ Touchdown ➤

We've been teasing and playing, deliberately avoiding the clitoris, in an effort to get her absolutely yearning to be touched there. There will be a time when the right place to touch is the clitoris. When her desire is maxed out and her clitoris is aching to be touched, it's a go. You want to select her favored spot. As we have written, most women's favorite spot on their clitoris is the upper left quadrant (this is her left, as in her left hand), but we have seen a number of women who prefer their upper right quadrant or even their lower quadrants, so you cannot make assumptions. If you are unsure, start with the upper left unless she tells you otherwise. Anyhow, when you do get to the clitoris, you want to start touching her right away on her favorite, most turned-on area. In order to do so, you will have to move her hood out of the way.

➤ Retracting the Hood ➤

All women's genitals are shaped differently. This goes for the hood of the clitoris, too. Some hoods are quite thick, and others are quite thin. Some women's clitorises are totally buried under the hood, and other women have practically no hood at all. Before even starting to touch the clitoris, it is an excellent idea to take visual inventory of the area—to determine the lay of the land, so to speak. Determine what type of hood she has and how her clitoris relates to the hood geographically. Pull back on the hood area to see what it will take to be able to freely touch all parts of the clitoral head.

Figures 15 and 16 illustrate how to pull back on the hood with either your right or left hand. You will probably want to use your dominant hand to both retract the hood and stroke the clitoris. Press the meaty part of your thumb against the side of the hood and pull up. You want to expose as much of her clitoris as you can. Until you've learned her preferences, use the training cycle (Chapter 3) to ask questions as you vary the amount of pressure you apply. Most women like firm pressure here and can take more pressure than you may think. Whether her preferred touch is firm or light, remember that your touch must be sure and deliberate at all times—not tentative—even when you're pulling back on the hood. Pulling back the clitoral hood with the thumb of your stroking hand in just the right way is one of the most difficult and important techniques to master, and it is one that we want our male students to learn well early on. It is so important because it frees up your second hand for other activities.

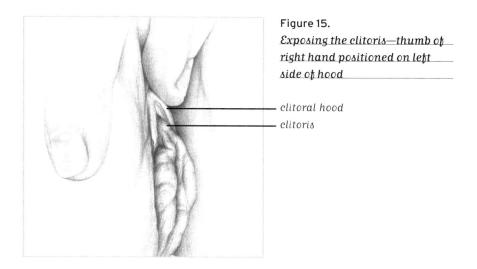

Figure 15.
Exposing the clitoris—thumb of right hand positioned on left side of hood

clitoral hood
clitoris

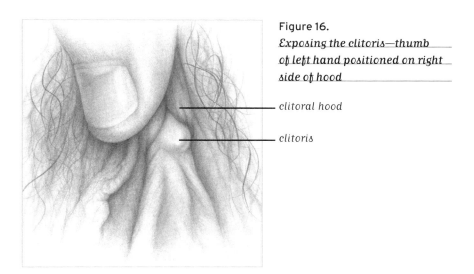

Figure 16.
Exposing the clitoris—thumb of left hand positioned on right side of hood

clitoral hood
clitoris

Once you know how to showcase the clitoris by pulling back the hood, put some lubricant on the tip of your index or middle finger and stroke the clitoris. The stroke is almost a pinching motion between the finger and the thumb that is holding back the hood (you are essentially moving your finger against your stationary thumb). I like to start with a very short stroke on her favorite clitoral quadrant. The pressure and the speed I use will depend on what I know about my subject and upon how I feel at the moment. With my full attention on her, I will know just what feels best. I will give her one stroke at a time if we are practicing feeling the first stroke. Each time I start to pleasure a woman, even the same woman, I do not follow a specific plan.

There is, however, a specific way to hold your hand and finger. Even when you retract the hood, the upper portions or quadrants of the clitoris are still usually partially covered by the hood, especially at the beginning, before the clitoris is fully engorged. You will have to dig your finger under the hood to get to the upper quadrants. Hook your index finger under the hood, probably at an angle, to allow you access to the proper quadrant (see Figure 17). If you are right handed, to get to the upper left quadrant, you can tilt your wrist as if looking at your watch.

Figure 17.
Hook right index finger under hood to fully expose upper left quadrant of clitoris

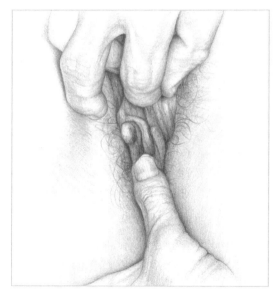

In general, unless you are practicing the one-stroke-at-a-time technique, use continuous short strokes on her favorite spot. For now, don't change the type of stroke you use. The number of strokes you give her at first will depend on her response to your stimulation.

⇒ Stroking the Lower Clitoris ⇐

Here is a fun and easy stroke that most women find quite pleasurable. Instead of digging your finger under the hood, place the finger at the lower part of her clitoris where it is attached to the inner lips. You can touch or stroke this area on both sides simultaneously or on one side at a time. Of course, you have a little lubricant on your fingertip. Lightly stroke with an up-and-down motion, moving to the beat of the music, if you like. You can even use single strokes to continue her training to feel that very first stroke. Let her know that you are rubbing at the bottom of her clitoris or even a little below and off of it. In this way she will not think that you are failing to find her upper left quadrant but will know that you are touching her exactly where you want to.

This stroke is very easy to do as there is no hood in the way, even without your having to retract it. We have worked with a number of women who have hoods that are either fully attached to their clitorises or partly attached and are therefore impossible to retract. These women (as well as women whose hoods are easily retractable) usually enjoy a lot of pleasurable sensitivity in the boundary between the upper portions of their labia minora and their clitoris. It is also an effective stroke for untrained women (as we will describe in the next chapter), who at first may like this type of touch even more than being stimulated directly on their spot.

⇒ Placement of Your Second Hand ⇐

See Figure 8 in the previous chapter (page 85) for a recommended position for your second hand. Confidently grasp her buttocks cheeks, and place your thumb firmly yet politely at the base of her introitus. The job of this thumb is to feel the strength of the contractions in her PC muscle, which encircles the vaginal and anal openings in the shape of a figure eight.

This hand placement allows most women to feel they are being taken care of, which increases their ability to relax. It allows you to sense if she starts to tense her muscles and lift her torso, at which moment a friendly reminder to sink into your hand will usually be enough to get her to relax again. This position also makes the second thumb available to stimulate her genitals in coordination with your primary stroking hand. You can move this thumb up and down along the introitus or inner lips as you continue to stroke the clitoris.

If through her body language (or verbally) she invites you into her vagina, your thumb can easily slip inside and stroke as you continue to rub the clitoris with your primary hand. Penetration should not be forced, but if she bids you inside you can use your thumb to press downward with the pad or press upward with the nail area. Make sure that you keep your nails short. Do whatever feels best, and always stay in communication with your partner about her preferences. Sometimes I will insert my thumb as far as it will go, press down firmly but not too hard, and keep it there as I continue to stroke the clitoris with my primary hand. Read *The Illustrated Guide to Extended Massive Orgasm* for more descriptions of how to penetrate the vagina with your fingers.

Alternatively, you may want to use the second hand to pull back on the hood, as we described earlier. This allows good access to the clitoris, but you lose the ability to judge the strength of her contractions. You can try this method to start a session or if you are unable to pull back the hood with the thumb of your stroking hand. You can now easily engorge and expose the clitoris, and then later place your second hand under her buttocks to feel her contractions.

There are times when I may put the index or middle finger of my second hand on her introitus, closer to the clitoris, without using the rest of that hand (see Figure 9 on page 86). This allows me to feel the strength of her contractions while causing as little distraction as possible. Then I may use that finger to stroke the introitus as I continue to stroke the clitoris. All of this depends on how I feel—on my response to what is occurring in her body. Once a woman invites your hand inside her vagina, your fingers will practically be sucked in. You can then add more fingers if you like. This usually happens after she has been pleasured for a while. Continue to stroke her clitoris as you play inside her vagina.

∿

The next chapter offers advanced tips for utilizing these techniques on both trained and untrained women. It also describes additional strokes and hand positions that will boost your creativity in taking your partner to heights of sensual delight.

CHAPTER 6

Advanced Tips
for Creating Orgasms

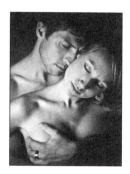

*I*n this chapter we will go into more detail about how to take control of your partner's level of tumescence. We will describe how to relate to a partner who is totally new to being pleasured in this way, and how to relate to one whose body is already trained in the art of receiving pleasure. With the same type of touch, one person may soar beyond the atmosphere and another may barely get off the ground. We will describe additional strokes and positions that can increase your ability to be that special lover. By staying true to your integrity, learning to engage your full attention, and practicing the techniques outlined in this book, you will be able to take anyone anyplace.

⇒ Control and Confidence ⇐

The concept of control has a negative connotation in our society. Who wants to be labeled a control freak? The fact is, if someone is in the position of giving pleasure to another, then the more he or she has control of the experience, the more the pleasure recipient can surrender and the higher they can go. Like all things, control is neither good nor bad in and of itself. When it comes to the production of pleasure, being in control is a good thing.

Ironically, the best way to be in control of any situation is to be in agreement with the way things are, rather than trying to force things to be the way you think they ought to be. As soon as a person is out of agreement with any aspect of reality, he or she is no longer in control. The sooner a person gets back into agreement with things, the sooner he or she will be back in control. We often compare this notion to the phenomenon of driving a car on an icy road and going into a skid. As long as you fight what is going on by trying to turn the steering wheel in the direction opposite that of the skid, you will lose control of the car. The only way to get back into control is to get into agreement with the skid—to turn the wheel in the same direction that the skid is taking you.

How do these twin concepts of agreement and control relate to pleasuring someone? It is about having your attention on your partner and noticing what they are feeling and which direction they are going, either up or down, and then responding to the situation with just the right amount of force, retreat, or leverage. It is about approving of and getting into agreement with the responses in your partner's body and knowing when is the right moment to take them to a new level.

In order to be in control of the situation, you have to know how to deal with all kinds of possible resistances, which we hope you have read about and digested from our previous chapters. This is where studying and practicing the art of giving pleasure translates into increased confidence. The more confidence a person feels and displays, the better position they will be in to control events as they occur. They will know what to do, or at least will have some clarity about what the next right move might be. They will be in the driver's seat and thus able to respond to all kinds of challenges. They will be a step or two ahead in the struggle for control and will masterfully be able to take their partner to new, desirable places.

Once the pleasure recipient surrenders and allows you to take control of her or his nervous system, it becomes that much easier to direct the experience. A person can gain confidence from pleasuring someone who surrenders easily. This is part of the training we offer through our books, classes, and DVDs. A man who learns how fun and easy it can be to give a woman orgasmic pleasure will become dedicated to and enthusiastic about the proposition of doing so. He will have enough confidence to recognize the difference between real and faked orgasmic responses. Of course, this is really only possible with manual stimulation. A penis inserted into a vagina is not a reliable indicator of the woman's orgasm, only its own.

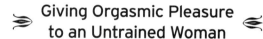

Giving Orgasmic Pleasure to an Untrained Woman

The intensity and duration of a woman's orgasm will vary depending on whether she is familiar or unfamiliar with the sort of intense, focused stimulation we advocate—that is, on whether she is "trained" or "untrained." It can be fun and rewarding to give pleasure to an untrained woman. Her response will depend on her natural ability to receive orgasmic pleasure, her acceptance of the ideas of instant and extended orgasm, whether she has masturbated this way, whether she uses a vibrator (usually counterproductive), and how relaxed and surrendered you can make her feel.

It is almost always a good idea to talk first—to explain what you plan to do, how you would like her to respond to your requests, and how she can modify what you are doing by asking for what she desires. Remember that the goal of each session or "date" can be different. Sometimes you may agree that you will work on causing her to feel the very first stroke with more intensity, as this book emphasizes, and at other times you may want to work on extending the orgasm. Think of these as training sessions; therefore, setting aside specific time to enjoy the practice and going over the landscape before getting there are recommended. If you want to practice heightening orgasmic sensation, not all of your dates have to be training sessions, but it is a good idea to treat at least some of them as such, or at least a portion of some of them.

Sometimes a person is so new to this information that it is best to first seduce them into really wanting the experience, even if they say they wish to try. Then when you do get them into bed, don't necessarily expect them to feel the first stroke with orgasmic intensity. Early on, the goal is to help them relax as much as possible and to have fun with them. Be playful and enjoy their doubts and resistances. Their doubts are actually a covert kind of resistance; instead of just saying no to you, they are saying they are unsure of themselves or do not know if they can do it. Or maybe, once the touching has started, they move their bodies a lot, which is a sign (among many possible signs) that they are not feeling as much as they could. You have to play with these doubts by first noticing them and then handling them skillfully. The best way to treat most people is with kindness and slow, deliberate training—or what Vera sometimes calls "baby steps." Gently coax them into going just a little farther than they expected to, and reward them for taking the leap. These baby steps will add up once they see what is possible, and soon you will be able to go full speed ahead.

Whether you're delivering the first stroke or any subsequent stroke, the principle is the same: The recipient needs to place her or his full attention on the part of their body that is being touched, and they need to focus on enjoying the sensation with all of their ability. When one is receiving many strokes, the best way to continue feeling is to imagine that each stroke in a series is the only one, and to focus on feeling that one stroke as intensely as possible. Sometimes the strokes happen so fast that it becomes difficult to separate each one, yet the goal remains the same: to feel as much as you can. When people ask us how to have an extended orgasm, we often answer, "One stroke at a time."

Because of my reputation and confidence, I can often seduce a woman who may be new to this experience into feeling her pussy and her clitoris before we even begin touching. She knows that I know what I am doing, and she knows that although she is vulnerable I will not take advantage of the situation for anything besides producing pleasure in her body. She feels safe having another woman, Vera, in the room, a woman who is also focusing a lot of attention on her. She knows we are there for her pleasure and also that we are enjoying ourselves. She can feel our intention. Because we have talked first, she knows there will be few surprises, and she can learn to relax into the experience.

My point here is to emphasize (again) the importance of knowing your craft and being skillful. The more confident the pleasure giver is—in a kind way rather than a smug or threatening way—the more the recipient can focus on pleasure and the less they need to focus on protecting themselves. Often, a first-time pleasure recipient will feel nervous. This is another reason to talk first and assist them in putting their nervous energy into their genitals rather than into their head, stomach, throat, or wherever. Nervousness is just a form of energy, and it can be used positively or can cause problems, depending on how it is handled. We often tell our students that they can convert their nervous energy into orgasmic energy. If you were to ignore your partner's nervousness and sweep it under the rug, it would show up later and prevent more pleasure. Yet if you address the edginess, you can use it to create more intimacy and more sensation. Keep reminding her to send that energy to her genitals until you notice that it is gone. It is up to the giver of pleasure to make sure that the energy is channeled properly and functionally.

Sometimes you can feel the heat of this nervous energy where it becomes stuck at some point in her body, often in the throat area. Review the sections "Feel the Heat" and "Point-and-Feel Orgasm" in Chapter 4 for a description of how to help the pleasure recipient move energy into her genitals. These "preliminary" activities will help her to relax, trust your ability to sense what's going on within her, focus on her own pleasure, and release her nervousness and fear.

⪼ The Position ⪻

Before getting into position, I like to make sure there is a large towel under where our bodies will be, the pillows are aligned against the headboard or wall, and I have easy access to lubricant and "do towels" (little hand towels or wash cloths used to wipe away lubricant and ejaculate after the activity is finished). There can be a pillow available to place under her thigh when she gets into position. I also like to have music playing and water or another beverage within arm's reach, preferably with a straw so I can administer a few sips without her having to get up or move. Make sure the phone or a knock on the bedroom door will not disturb you. These preparations are useful even if your partner is experienced.

One can use a number of different positions to manually pleasure a woman's genitals. Our favorite is the perpendicular sitting position (see Figure 18). It usually works best if the pleasure giver gets into position first. Making sure that the pillows are firm against your back, straighten out the bath towel and invite her to lie down at a ninety degree angle to you so that her head is toward the side of the bed and on the side of your dominant hand—your right side if you're right-handed, or your left side if you're left-handed. What follows are instructions for a right-handed person; reverse them if you're left-handed. Place your right leg over her abdomen and your left leg under her legs. Make sure her legs are bent and spread as far apart as possible. Place the extra pillow under her outside leg for support; position her inside leg comfortably over your left thigh. Your right leg is bent over her abdomen with your knee facing upward so you can rest your arm on it.

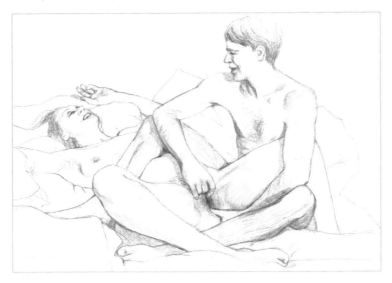

Figure 18. *Sitting position on bed (what's depicted is for a right-handed pleasure giver)*

You can modify this position by sitting Indian style or using a chair with the woman still perpendicular to you (*The Illustrated Guide to Extended Massive Orgasm* depicts many positions); however, the one described above is the best we have found. It allows both of you to remain comfortable for an extended period of time, it provides excellent visibility of her genitals, and face-to-face communication is easy. We recommend using adequate lighting, especially direct light on her genitals, so that you can see what you are doing. Some women do not like to have bright lights on during intimate activity; if this is the case she can always wear a blindfold or lightly position the edge of a pillow over her eyes if that would make her feel better. With the lighting focused directly on her genitals you won't have the problem of it shining in her face. We have found that after a number of times of doing this with the lights on, almost everyone gives up their old preference for doing it in the dark.

Sometimes I will ask the woman to lie down first. Then I can stand at the side of the bed and talk to her some more to get her to relax. I can squeeze or rub her feet and sensually stroke her legs toward her crotch, coaxing her to start feeling. Then I climb over her and get into position. I readjust her body, pulling her as close to me as I can while staying perpendicular. I make sure her legs are bent and that I can easily place my hands on her genitals.

⇒ Challenges ⇐

Whether they're trained or untrained, some women who are quite overweight will have body fat in their thigh area that obscures the view of their genitals. If your partner is easily orgasmic this won't prevent you from sensing her pleasure, but it may present more difficulty if you're pleasuring someone who is new to these techniques. You can still separate the legs with both hands to see the genitals. Unfortunately, once your hands are removed it will become difficult to see them. When you start stroking, you will have to use your sense of touch. During pauses and breaks, you can always separate the folds of flesh again to view the beautiful crotch and to observe the engorgement and other signs of orgasm.

Any of the resistances we've already discussed are likely to occur when someone is just beginning to tap into her sensual potential. She may resist by trying to help you out (moving her hips), or she may have a sensitive clitoris that cannot be touched directly. She will probably use any chance she gets to test you. Prepare for the worst (even though you can hope for better) by re-reading the sections in this book on handling resistances.

We have heard from a number of men whose partners, new or established, did not like the idea of just lying there and being the recipient of all the plea-sure. (Of course, there are also many women out there who would love to be the recipient of this kind of pleasure.) These women thought that they would perhaps owe the man the same treatment, or they felt too exposed—two types of feelings that were forms of resistance that prevented them from being at total effect. Men, if you are in this predicament, you will have to learn how to seduce your partner into wanting to receive more pleasure. You will have to determine what her specific resistances are and play with them. This can be a fun game, and we recommend reading our book *To Bed or Not to Bed* for fur-ther edification on the topic.

⇒ Touching ⇐

So now you are both in position. You can tell her that you are going to touch her body with your hands and arms. If you have not done so already, find out if there are any places on her body that are off-limits and what parts of her body are most responsive to touch—for example, whether she likes her nip-ples played with or her neck caressed. Remember to use a touch that you en-joy; the goal as pleasure giver is to touch for your own pleasure. Remind her to let you know if she is enjoying the touches using simple comments such as "That feels good" or "Yes, I like that." It's very important to keep your finger-nails short and trimmed of any sharp edges, and also to keep your hands as soft as possible by using moisturizer regularly.

When I'm working with a student I am fully clothed; whether you are fully or partially nude is a matter to discuss beforehand with your partner. You can start by playing with her nipples if she likes that, often using a little lubricant. You can rub them lightly one at a time with your wrist. I love women's legs so I will often lightly stroke them. You can use any kind of stroke that feels good to you—large circles, small circles, up and down, full palm, fingertips, the back of your hand, your fingernails, or whatever. Most women prefer a light touch. At this point you can start teasing her genitals by moving toward them from the thigh and then backing away, and then returning even closer the next time. You can let her know how great it feels to you to stroke her thighs, what soft skin or nice muscle tone she has—whatever it is about her that you find pleasing.

At some point you will want to spread her labia, exposing her introitus and clitoris to get a better view, as normally the two inner labia are touching one another, kind of sealing up the area. You can also feel the heat more strongly when the lips are spread apart. Let her know how pretty and pink her pussy is; women really like to hear that. Don't shower her with empty compliments, of course. Be honest. You can always find something to appreciate.

If she is still at all nervous, ask her again to relocate that energy to her genital area, assisting her by moving your hand from the top of her body downward toward her genitals, never touching her but hovering close enough to feel any heat or energy she is producing. Once the heat is emanating from her genitals you may have to go back and spread her labia again. This is usually fun for the recipient as she is receiving full visual attention on her most private area. It is important to acknowledge how much you enjoy the sight. Describe all the nuances you notice, such as different colors, and describe and compliment any engorgement or bodily lubricant. You can tell her how wonderful she smells, too, if you enjoy her fragrance. Now that she is opened you can put some lubricant on her genitals, or you can go back to teasing the area by lightly running your hand or wrist over or through her pubic hair (see Figure 19 on the next page) or by playing some more with her thighs or her lower abdomen, which is also sensitive.

You want her to feel everything you are doing. Place your full attention on her, and be deliberate in your actions even though this is a go-with-the-moment experience rather than one that's been fully planned in advance. Stay in communication with your partner and look at her face occasionally for tips about how she is appreciating your attentions. If she isn't enjoying things, find out what is going on. Is she apprehensive? Staying in her head too much? By talking with her, you often will be able to help her feel more, get back into her body, and have more fun. You can tell her that it is okay to enjoy herself and to smile.

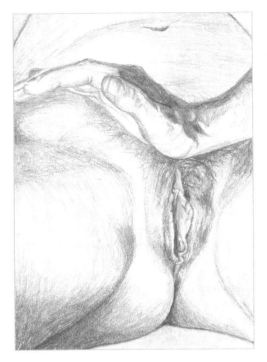

Figure 19.
Playing with her
pubic hair

At some point, once there is more heat coming from her genitals, you can hold your hand slightly above her clitoris and ask her to feel your attention and to feel the closeness of your hand. Use the many techniques we've outlined in earlier chapters to play around the clitoral area itself before making direct contact. As always, let her know what you are going to do before doing it so that she will not be kept wondering or feel threatened.

When you are ready to put lubricant onto her genitals, let her know that you will be doing so. Remember that it is more than okay to be lustful and to enjoy touching her genitals during the act of spreading lube. Instruct her to feel each stroke. Again, the best way to insure that she does so is for you to take as much pleasure as you can with your fingers. Linger over any part that you especially enjoy touching. Avoid getting lubricant on the hood of the clitoris.

⤜ Finding the Right Pressure ⤛

Once you're ready to make contact with the clitoris, tell her what you are going to do right before doing it; for example, say, "I'm going to pull back your hood with my thumb now." Use any of the techniques we've described for doing so. You may use a firm pressure to retract the hood, but make sure that your partner likes the pressure you're using. Avoid exerting excessive pressure with your finger under the hood; you do not want her to become defensive or feel any pain. On the other hand, it can be difficult to dig your finger under the hood without using pressure. The more you practice, the better you will be at feeling your way through the process.

Some women like a lot of pressure, but most prefer less. Many of our women students complain that their partners use too much force on their clitorises. We ask them if they have told their lovers of their preferences, and most say they have but that their partner still uses too much pressure. So in reality they have not communicated their preferences to their partners explicitly enough. They tried once or twice and then decided to find their partners at fault or inadequate rather than communicating precisely how they want to be touched. Furthermore, a person who is unfamiliar with a woman's genitals and whose touch is tentative or lacking in confidence will often get a negative response no matter what sort of touch or amount of pressure he uses. Again, it is a matter of her surrendering to whatever he is doing, and the less she trusts his attentions the less pleasure will result.

Once you've selected which clitoral quadrant to touch based on the location of your partner's favorite spot (see "Touchdown," in Chapter 5), make sure your first touch is deliberate and that you feel it as intensely as you can, which should help your partner feel it as well. The goal is for your partner to experience orgasmic pleasure with that first stroke. You can put your finger right over her clitoris after exposing it and kind of hover there, waiting for her to place her total attention on her clitoris before you begin to touch it. You can tease her by saying that you are very close, but that you are going to wait until she is totally ready.

Some newcomers are unable to feel much on the first stroke. If this is the case, it may be a good idea to deliver a few strokes directly to her favorite spot and then take a break. Remove your hands, talk some, and start again. Now try the one-stroke-at-a-time sequence. We have found that women who use vibrators often have a problem feeling at first because they are so used to the artificially intense sensations delivered by those contraptions. Women who are serious about increasing their orgasmic capacity will have to become more dedicated to using their own hands to practice instead of relying on their vibrator.

⋙ Crotch Diving ⋘

In general, it is a good idea to approach your partner's genitals slowly rather than diving right in, an approach that we call crotch diving. This rule is not carved in stone; there will be some times when crotch diving is appropriate. However, by slowly approaching and teasing your partner (or yourself, for that matter), you create desire. You want to make it so that they are really craving and thirsting for your touch on their hot spots. To dive right in when a person is not quite ready and is not greedy for your touch indicates that you don't have your full attention on them. This is especially true for an untrained woman, who is more likely than a trained woman to need some time to feel safe enough to surrender.

This also goes for playing with a man's penis. Take your time. You do not have to go straight for his member.

⋙ Instant-Orgasm Training ⋘

When we take on new women as students, we want to teach them how to have an EMO. This includes the ability to be in orgasm right away, without requiring a buildup of continual stroking. Toward that end, we ask them to do their homework, which consists of learning to feel their genitals without touching them and also touching themselves one stroke at a time while feeling as much as they can.

Learning to be instantly orgasmic is, of course, a process and usually doesn't happen overnight or in one session, although sometimes it does. The more a woman can focus her attention and approve of any pleasurable feelings, the more open she will be to experiencing even greater sensation the next time. She does not have to feel a whole lot at first, but simply to approve of any little sensation she notices. This is a fun path, and no matter how fast or slow a person travels along it, as long as she is progressing she will find it very gratifying.

⇒ Touching a Trained Woman ⇐

Giving pleasure to a woman who has trained her body to feel pleasure at the first stroke and who has experienced an EMO is a fun privilege. This type of woman no longer has to be trained to feel the first stroke because she has already graduated from that fundamental concept. Basically, though, the pleasure giver's task is pretty much the same as it is with an untrained woman. Start by touching her anywhere on her body. Remember to touch for your own pleasure, keep your full attention on her, lubricate her when ready, and expose her clitoris when it is time to begin stroking it. Do not be in a rush at any point during the preliminary activities, and enjoy and report all signs of pleasure you notice in her body.

When pleasuring a trained woman, you can usually increase the length of the peak to encompass many strokes before deliberately changing the stroke to bring her down. You still want to direct all of your attention to her so you can notice when it is time to peak. The period between peaks can be much shorter than it is with an untrained woman. Instead of removing your hands from her body and talking, you may just skip one beat and then start stroking again. As long as she perceives that you know what you're doing and are in control, she will go along with and take pleasure from most anything you do. She can surrender to any kind of stroke, whether it is a repetitive stroke directly on her favored spot, or whether you only touch her favorite spot every few strokes as you move your finger around her clitoris and the surrounding vicinity. She can respond pleasurably to a fast stroke, a slow stroke, firm pressure, or light pressure. It really doesn't matter what you do as long as you enjoy yourself and remain in control, which is another way of saying that you know what you are doing and everything you do is deliberate. Remember that control is synonymous with agreement, which means that you do not have to work hard to create an orgasm in a woman who is pleasured easily. All you have to do is stay conscious and avoid getting in the way of her orgasm. Once she has surrendered, she will go for her pleasure with all she has. You are there for the ride, occasionally peaking her or, if anything, keeping her back a little from going too high all at once. You can do this by taking her along a new path with your attention focused on where she is in her orgasmic cycle. The best thing you have to offer her is your pleasure in touching her. You do not have to force anything.

Just separating her inner lips is a real thrill. You will often notice contractions and the obvious joy she takes in receiving attention on her pussy. Exposing the genitals of a woman who takes pleasure in being pleasured is so wonderful and life-enhancing that this small act in itself is practically miraculous—yet it is also repeatable. It is ever so gratifying to slide your lubricated fingers over her inner labia and the rest of her genitals. We always use lubricant, even with women who have orgasms easily. Your fingers will notice the apparent and effortless joy she experiences when you're applying the lubricant. You can use different amounts of pressure along the introitus and up to the base of her clitoris, and you will often sense stronger and stronger contractions. You still have not touched the clitoral head directly and she is already having an orgasm. This is what all the practice and training have been about: to feel almost all sensations on one's genitals as provocatively delightful.

Now you can go directly to the clitoris or can play around for as long as you like and as long as the person receiving the attention is being gratified. This may depend in part on how much time you have. If you have a meeting to go to or kids to attend to, there may be a limit to how much teasing you indulge in. But once you touch the clitoris, it usually is a good idea to stay there and not go back to, say, the thigh, unless you are deliberately peaking your partner. Although we do not typically recommend crotch diving, on occasion when pressed for time and when pleasuring an easily orgasmic woman, we have gone deep-sea diving without any teasing. We just go for the clitoris with some lubricant, even inserting fingers right away if she so desires. Usually, however, we do not just dive in but instead play around using different pressures and touches.

Even when I am pleasuring Vera, I may keep my finger hovering over her clitoris and ask her to feel it. She will start having contractions. A person can always get better at being instantly orgasmic. All of the techniques we've described in this book can be implemented to cause her to feel that initial pleasure. The more one practices, the more pleasurable it becomes. One of our students remarked that just getting into position and placing my hands over

Vera's body produced a Pavlovian orgasmic response in Vera. It is fun to be creative here, and you can do anything that feels good to both of you.

≽ Ready, Set, Clitoris ≼

When I am ready to begin stroking her clitoral head I first get my hands into position. Sometimes I place my second (nonstroking) hand on her body before I place my stroking hand, and sometimes I place it afterward. Sometimes I slide both hands into position at the same time. With a trained woman it does not really matter what order you do things in as long as she knows that you know what you're doing. (See earlier chapters for ideas about placing your hands.) Especially take note of the best position for your stroking hand, with the thumb available to pull back on the clitoral hood and the index or middle finger available for stroking the head. The stroke is practically a pinching motion between finger and thumb—as if you were picking up a hundred-dollar bill. The thumb does not move, only the index or middle finger.

I typically go straight to the woman's favorite spot on her clitoris with a little lubricant on my index finger and give her a number of small up-and-down strokes there. Because I am trained and she is trained, we will know where that spot is. When you are pleasuring a woman who has been trained, listen to her when she tells you where her favorite spot is. As we have said, a great majority of women are most sensitive on the upper left quadrant, but we have found that the upper right quadrant is the most sensitive in about 10 percent of women. Do not argue by telling her that you've read that all women are most sensitive on the upper left quadrant of their clitoris. The whole clitoral head is covered with nerve endings and a person can be pleasured anywhere on it. By heeding her wishes you will remain in control and she can surrender to you more easily than if you were to argue. Once the clitoris becomes engorged it will not matter which part of it you stroke, as long as you keep feeling her pleasure and your own. Because her body is trained to feel every stroke, you can sense all contractions with your finger on the clitoris and with your second hand at the base of her introitus. Some women have stronger contractions than others, and on different days the same woman will experience different degrees of pleasure.

➣ The First Peak ➤

Repeated stroking will almost always engorge the clitoris to a much larger size than when you started. You can feel the clitoris getting harder and filling with blood. Be sure to tell your partner what you observe. Continue stroking as long as you sense that she is going higher in intensity and sensation. At some point you will realize that it is time to peak her—in other words, to deliberately bring her down. All you have to do is stop stroking and lift your finger off the clitoris. Before or as you do so, you might let her know that it is time for a break or that you are peaking her. Then take a good look at her genitals and describe how engorged and red her clitoris and labia have become.

After the first peak, put your finger back on her clitoris and begin stroking again. You can use the same kind of stroke as before, perhaps a little faster, or use a different one. We almost always have music playing during sensual activity, whether it is with students or just the two of us. It can be fun to kind of dance on your partner's clitoris to the beat of the music. If the music doesn't fit, you can go half-time or double-time. Learn to use music as a guide at times, but remember that you are in charge of the rhythm and must decide what is best at each moment.

➣ Different Strokes ➤

Once the clitoris is fully engorged, try moving your finger to different parts of the clitoris—place a few strokes on the upper left, a few strokes on the upper right, then on the lower left, lower right, upper middle, lower middle, return to upper left, and so on. You don't have to keep repeating the same sequence; you can move around on the clitoris at will, still stroking to the beat of the music. This strategy works really well once you have taken full control of her nervous system and she has surrendered completely. She knows that you know where her favorite spot is and that you will stroke it when you so desire, and she will enjoy every move you make. I usually like to move my fingers pretty quickly when doing this type of stroke. I therefore like to have music with a fast beat for this portion of the session.

You can see here how important it is to be able to get off on that first stroke and to feel every stroke as if it were the one and only. Moving around the clitoris (and sometimes around other areas of her genitals) may also work on a less trained woman, but it will have a different effect. Instead of taking her up on a continuous run, she may come down when you move away from her spot. This gives her a chance to refocus and to feel your finger when it goes back to her favorite quadrant. We have noticed that when a woman is first starting her training, she often prefers not to receive too many consecutive strokes on her favorite spot.

➤ More Positions ◄

One of my favorite hand positions is with the base of my palm on the woman's lower abdomen or pubic area and my index or middle finger on her clitoris (see Figure 20). This stroke is best to utilize after the clitoris has become engorged and is more visible and accessible, which means you do not have to use your thumb or other hand to retract the hood. Hold your hand steady, or rhythmically press your palm downward, while moving your finger on her clitoris at will. Place all of your attention on the fun sensations in your finger. I like to use a light, gliding kind of stroke here, as though I were skating on her clitoris (no double axels). She is in the throes of her orgasm and it is sheer fun. You can use this stroke on some untrained women, too.

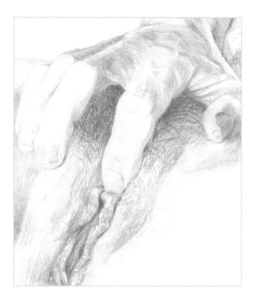

Figure 20.
Pressure on mons
while stroking clitoris

Sometimes I will use my middle finger on Vera's clitoris as we are lying side by side next to each other (see Figure 21). In this position, I may use my thumb to press on her pubic area, which pulls the hood back to some degree, while I stroke her clitoris. I can play with various levels of pressure with my thumb or the base of my palm (see Figure 22). This position should mainly be used by folks who are trained and know what they are doing, as it prevents the giver from seeing the receiver's genitals. The good part is that our faces are close together and we can kiss and talk easily; it is a little less technical and perhaps more romantic. The woman is also in a good position to play with her partner's penis. The pleasure giver can still put his second hand under her buttocks to feel the contractions. Instead of placing the thumb of my second hand at her introitus, I will use the middle finger of my second hand. It is also convenient in that we can be lying in bed and move to this position in no time flat, as opposed to having to rearrange the pillows and our bodies to get into a sitting position. If you're feeling lazy, this position can help you remember that what you're doing is fun and not work.

Figure 21. Side-by-side position (what's depicted is for a right-handed pleasure giver)

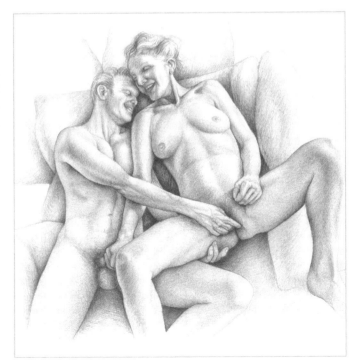

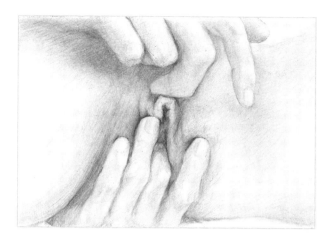

Figure 22. *Position of hands in side-by-side position*

➲ Fun or Work? ⋐

Speaking of fun versus work, anytime you are pleasuring someone you don't want it to feel like hard work, no matter what kind of stroke you are using. When you are learning your craft you may at first have some difficulty getting the hood pulled back with the thumb of your stroking hand, or trying to stay on her spot, or doing some of the other techniques we describe. This may feel like work, and you are in training, so it is training work. Still, if it becomes too painful or too hard, do something different, like pulling back her hood with your other hand, or find an easier stroke. Once you get the techniques down pat giving pleasure must be only about pleasure. If it feels like hard work at any time then you must take a break. It is also time for a break when any part of your body, whether your stroking hand or your leg or your back, is cramping or hurting or distracting you in any way. Switch to a different position, or otherwise adjust things by moving a pillow or the like. If your hand is cramping it may be a sign that your partner is tensing her body. Again, taking a break and talking about relaxing can go a long way toward making things better.

➲ The Surround Stroke ⋐

I like this stroke a lot (see Figure 23 on the next page). It is best done in the perpendicular sitting position. Place the index and middle fingers of your

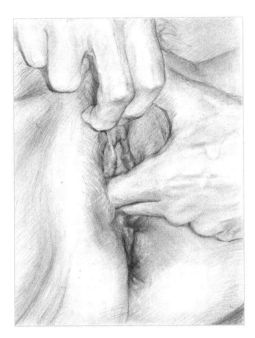

Figure 23.
Surround stroke

nonstroking (nondominant) hand inside the woman's vagina, finger pads facing up. This gives you access to the region on the front side of the vaginal wall typically called the G-spot. The thumb of this hand is then free to circle up to her mons area, where it can pull back on the hood to expose the clitoris. Then the fingers of your stroking (dominant) hand can play with her clitoris in whatever way you want to without the thumb having to simultaneously retract the hood. The fingers of your nonstroking hand can massage the G-spot or other pleasurable areas in her vagina if you insert them deeply, or they can play with her labia if you barely insert them. Most of your attention will still be directed to her clitoris, but the second hand is making things easier by allowing you to massage the clitoral roots (located on the G-spot) from inside. This stroke is best done after your partner has been pleasured for some time, as you don't want to insert any fingers into her vagina until she is ready for it. And the clitoris will be easier to stroke in this position after it has engorged.

We have just described how to pleasure all kinds of women, from nonorgasmic to extremely orgasmic. Most fall somewhere in between. Almost all women, even very orgasmic ones, want to have better orgasms. And many men want to give their lovers this gift. By reading and rereading this chapter and practicing what you have read, you will be on the right path to reaching those goals.

The next chapter offers details about how to peak both women and men of all kinds of orgasmic capacity. With your partner's newfound ability to feel instantly, she or he will find a renewed appreciation for being peaked. Each new peak brings a chance to refeel that first stroke in its entirety.

CHAPTER 7

The Pleasure of Peaking

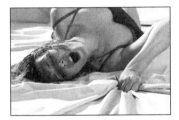

*T*hroughout this book we have mentioned peaking, which involves deliberately reducing the level of pleasurable or orgasmic intensity so that one can peak and hopefully go to a higher level with the next stroke or series of strokes. Some of you may already be fairly adept at peaking yourself and/or your partner. Because it is probably the most important ingredient in extending orgasmic pleasure (the "E" in EMO), we thought it proper to fully address how, when, and why to peak your partner. We've also included a section on peaking yourself.

Peaking is probably the last skill at which our students become fully proficient, but anyone can start using the technique early in their sensuality education. The key word, again, is "practice." It takes some time to become a master at peaking. The ability to be instantly orgasmic is beneficial here, as each new peak presents a new opportunity to feel the first stroke with as much of your attention as you can.

⪢ Slowing Down and Taking Breaks ⪡

As Milan Kundera writes in his novel *Slowness,* "Everything is composed, confected, artificial, everything is staged, nothing is straightforward, or in other words, everything is art; in this case; the art of prolonging the suspense, better yet; the art of staying as long as possible in a state of arousal."

And, later, "The haste that loses them that sweet slowness, both of them instantly see as an error, but I do not believe that this is any surprise to Madame de T., I think rather that she knew the error to be unavoidable, bound to occur, that she expected it, and for that reason she planned the interlude in the pavilion *a ritardando* to brake, to moderate, the foreseeable and foreseen swiftness of events so that, when the third stage arrived, in a new setting, their adventure might bloom in all its splendid slowness."

The novel continues, "By slowing the course of their night, by dividing it into different stages, each separate from the next, Madame de T. has succeeded in giving the small span of time accorded them the semblance of a marvelous little architecture, of a form. Imposing form on a period of time is what beauty demands, but so does memory. For what is formless cannot be grasped, or committed to memory. Conceiving their encounter as a form was especially precious for them, since their night was to have no tomorrow and could be repeated only through recollection."

And, finally, "In existential mathematics, that experience takes the form of two basic equations; the degree of slowness is directly proportional to the intensity of memory; the degree of speed is directly proportional to the intensity of forgetting."

How can we relate this idea of "slowness" to pleasure? The answer, it seems, is to create a "form," as Kundera calls it—an intentional, defined encounter. We can do this by taking breaks during the sensual episode. The slow and deliberate creation of the experience will benefit our efforts to grow more conscious and aware of our sensuality.

By taking breaks you create spaces—and therefore forms—in which to experience the sensual activity in a more defined way. In this way the experience will not be like a run-on sentence. It will be a series of short, well-defined statements. Breaking the episode into small intervals will create a better memory of the experience. It will provide an opportunity for both participants to "swallow" the pleasure. It will allow partners to be ready for the next short cycle. It will help the pleasure recipient feel one stroke at a time. It will result in an instant orgasm. It will lead to an extended massive orgasm.

Taking breaks doesn't mean going down all the way to the beginning after each break. It is different from a multiple orgasm, which is like a series of crotch sneezes. Rather, you start each cycle from a higher point than you started the previous cycle. Each cycle does not have to last a certain amount of time. Sometimes, if it feels right to do so, you may continue for a longer cycle. But be aware that most people tend to err on the too-long side. We think it is more fun to have shorter cycles, take more breaks, and restart when the desire builds again.

Working with students, we sometimes divide the session into different segments. Recently, we were training a man to give pleasure to his girlfriend. We didn't follow our usual routine, in which I first demonstrate on the woman by teasing her genitals, then lubricating her genitals, eventually getting to her clitoris with some stimulating strokes, and then handing her off to her partner. Instead, I showed him how to tease her genitals and then had him do it. Then I lubricated her all over, still teasing her but not yet touching her clitoris, wiped her off, and then had him do the same. Next, I got back in the saddle and showed him how to stroke her clitoris. I then handed her off to her partner so he could replicate my strokes. This sequence allowed him to pick things up much faster, so now we will use this teaching technique in all of our sessions with men who want to learn how to give women great pleasure.

We split up the sessions with our female students in a similar fashion. We may first talk to our student in the living room. Then we may go to the bedroom, where I demonstrate on Vera while the student watches and feels her own genital pleasure. Then I will play with and stimulate the student's body. For another cycle, we may go into another room and give her a peak on the massage table, and then take her back into the bedroom for some more pleasure.

This divides the experience into individual segments, allowing her to develop a better memory of the encounter. For each cycle we expect her to focus all of her available attention on her genitals and on her orgasmic sensations. Because the orgasm is continuous, although divided into discrete segments, she can start each cycle from a higher place. She can get used to starting higher and feeling more intensely. Then, at the next session, she remembers how she was able to start orgasming and feeling strong sensations from the get-go. It is a way of improving her ability to become instantly orgasmic.

We tell you about our teaching strategies because the same training principles apply to any sensual encounter. Especially when a lover, whether the giver or receiver of pleasure, is new to these techniques, the rule of thumb is to break events down, take them slowly, and create distinct little episodes, or "forms."

⇒ Specific Frames ⇐

Another great training tool is for partners to describe to each other some specific "frames" that each one recalls from the session. Specific frames are definable memories, comparable to a single frame from a film. Imagine watching a movie you enjoy and pressing the pause button at a particularly beautiful or interesting camera shot to linger on that single, still moment. In your conversations with your partner following a sensual encounter, describe to each other that kind of memory. The more specific detail you use in your description, the more turn-on you will create and the more pleasurable sensation you will feel. When someone relates an event from a very specific and detailed frame of reference, the person listening will feel like they were actually there. That is partially how turn-on can be created.

In the book *I Am a Strange Loop,* author Douglas Hofstadter writes about how his friend described a trip to Europe in such fine, specific detail that years later Hofstadter thought it was he himself who'd gone on that trip. He actually argued with his friend about which of them had really taken the trip.

This technique is very valuable if you want to learn to feel more and to be more conscious. One of the best ways to remember a specific frame is to verbally acknowledge a pleasurable moment while it is occurring. What you are really remembering is one single stroke at one single point in time and the precise sensation it creates in your body. Describing specific strokes greatly aids the process of becoming instantly orgasmic. As we have written, ongoing verbal appreciation is extremely important to remaining in present time and to allowing a person to go higher after they have "swallowed" a certain amount of pleasure. The recollection of this wonderful moment further increases one's consciousness and enjoyment of it. It is like getting two fun moments for the price of one.

To recap, the combination of dividing sessions into parts or segments, even into individual strokes, and verbalizing one's appreciation of these fun moments, both during the encounter and again later, is a great tool for feeling more on the first stroke and any strokes that follow.

Keeping a Pleasure Journal

Here's another teaching technique we use that can be easily incorporated into your sensual play with your partner. Our students keep a journal of their activities with us and often read journal entries from earlier sessions aloud to us. When the journal is filled with specific frames of intense pleasure, the simple act of reading aloud causes our female students to become easily turned on and begin to feel pleasurable sensations. When they write in generalities, no matter how well they have written, the effect is dramatically lessened, in direct proportion to the loss of specificity. Male students who are learning to give IOs and EMOs also gain skill much more quickly when they speak and write in specifics versus in generalities. With men, it is not so much that they turn themselves on, but that the effect of their words on the female teacher (or partner) can be beneficial to the ensuing session. To increase the passion in your relationship with your lover, consider keeping separate journals of your sensual encounters and reading your journal entries aloud to each other. Whether or not you keep a journal, learning how to speak and write about your sensual experiences with great specificity will promote your ability to notice, to appreciate, and to keep your attention on your partner (when you're the pleasure giver) and on your own pleasure (when you're the recipient).

Learning to speak about pleasure is contraindicated in our society, where a pain-oriented way of talking and thinking is the norm. Notice how often people talk about their painful or negative experiences. Even having sex or enjoying sensual pleasure is difficult for some. Some people still think of sexual pleasure as sinful. Besides just getting our students to talk, we have to constantly prod them to be more specific. The better their journals become, the better they are able to express themselves while receiving and giving pleasure. When a person is relating an event from the past in great detail, it feels like you are virtually there. You become integrated with that pleasurable moment and are able to live the experience yourself. To paraphrase Kundera, the degree of memory correlates with the degree of slowness. By slowing things down and isolating one specific moment, you create a treasure chest of memories.

⇒ Are You Peaking? ⇐

Knowing when to peak your partner and for how long is an art. You will develop and improve this skill over time, yet even as a novice you can still learn to peak someone at a suitable moment and for an appropriate length of time. There may be an exact best time to peak someone, but there are plenty of other points when it may be a fine time to peak someone. You can never know for sure when that exact point is. There are no bells or whistles or flashing lights that go on when you reach that precise moment. In general, however, it is better to peak someone too early than to peak them too late—or, as we tell our students, to quit them before they quit you. This means that as long as the pleasure is going smoothly, increasing, feeling wonderful, it is okay to keep stroking. But you want to stop stroking before the pleasure dips, before your partner goes down, before they slip even partially into their head and stop feeling as much as they were feeling before.

It will not make much difference in the long run if you quit someone a bit too early on any one peak. Maybe they could have gone a little higher for a little longer, but it is also true that they will be that much more eager to have you start stroking again. Sometimes you may be unsure whether it is the right time for a break. This uncertainty is actually a sign that it *is* time to take a break. If it were not the right time, you would not even be contemplating it. The person being rubbed on always has the option to ask you to keep stroking.

A number of years ago I was giving a woman pleasure and she started complaining that I was taking too many breaks and changing my stroke too often. (Changing strokes is another way of peaking someone that we will discuss in more detail shortly.) She never said, "Don't stop" or "Keep doing that" or even "This is so great." She only raised objections. I was deliberately peaking her because it felt like her arousal wasn't increasing, and I was giving her an opportunity to take it higher during the next round of stroking. I probably could have communicated better by informing her that I would keep the peaks short until she felt more. Whenever the person whom you are pleasuring finds you or your activities wrong, it is an indication that it may really be him or her who is not getting off as well as they might. I gave this student some longer peaks to see if that would make her happier, but that didn't work either. We were both fairly new to these techniques, so I did not take full control and she certainly did not surrender. Years later, when she had learned to have an EMO, I was able to give her longer peaks, yet at that point she would not have complained even if I had kept the peaks short.

So what do you do when a person asks you to keep stroking, yet you sense that they are not going higher? One of the things I do is to talk while I am still stroking. I tell them that I will keep stroking as long as I sense they are taking things higher, but I will take a break and perhaps stop altogether if they don't seem to be. I also tell them to keep acknowledging verbally, as that will help motivate me to continue.

⋙ Extending the Peak by Talking ⋘

You can keep extending the peak by talking your partner through it. Use this strategy when it seems clear that the pleasure recipient is still going for it, and you sense that they will soon stop feeling as much. Usually this is a good time to take a break or peak them by stopping or changing the stroke in some way. However, sometimes you may want them to broaden their ability to feel more intensely and to have longer periods of extended orgasm before you peak them by deliberately taking them down. You can do this by noticing and commenting on what is going on, and by expressing how you would like them to continue and respond to your verbal requests. Start by telling them that they are doing great and normally you would take a break but you want them to continue with this peak. Make some additional requests, such as "Keep feeling," "Take it up," "Just a little more," "Ten percent higher"—whatever seems like something they can accomplish. You can say something like, "This may be the last peak" or "I may only do a few more strokes" or "Feel these last ten strokes." Perform those strokes and then maybe say, "That's good. Now feel ten more," and so on.

Remember to let your partner know that they are doing well. Tell them to keep feeling or you will stop. You can say anything that comes into your head; for example, "I feel you," "I got you," or even "Yes" repeated over and over. It is also a good idea to keep them acknowledging their pleasure, as we've discussed throughout the book. Tell them that unless they continue verbalizing their appreciation, you are going to stop. You then must really stop if they refuse to acknowledge.

⪼ Attention Spans ⪻

We have noticed that a woman who has never received much direct clitoral stimulation has a rather small capacity for feeling pleasure there. It is like she has ADD and can only focus her attention for a brief period. She may start out by requiring only very short peaks indeed. The ability to focus one's attention for only a few strokes is quite normal at first. When you stroke a woman who is new to clitoral pleasuring, she may feel the first three or so strokes (as you can tell from the slight contractions in her introitus) yet may shut down by the fourth stroke. That means the fourth stroke was one too many; it would have been better to have given her only three strokes. The best thing to do is to tell her directly what you noticed—that she went away on the last stroke but you noticed that she felt the first three. Then tell her you will give her three strokes and stop, and that you will repeat this pattern for a number of cycles. She will probably continue to feel those three strokes. Next, tell her you will add a fourth stroke. By this time she will likely be able to feel all four strokes. You can also request that she continue to stay present and feel as intensely as possible as you add additional strokes. Keep progressing in these small increments, or baby steps, and soon your partner will be able to feel many strokes in a row.

If you give your partner too many strokes and sense her shutting down, it is a good idea to admit what happened. This will keep the communication up-to-date and honest and keep your side of the street clean, all of which will help you stay in control. If you keep stroking indiscriminately, it will be far more difficult to continue increasing your partner's level of arousal.

There are some women who even on the first attempt will be able to feel quite a few strokes. No strict formula exists, so, as always, the best policy is to remain at full attention. Then you can notice her capacity to respond and give her a more extended peak. Still, remember that it is generally better to peak her too soon than too late, so perhaps err on the side of caution. You can always quickly advance to longer peaks. Let her know that you can sense her feeling all of the strokes and that you will now add some more.

⮞ No Feeling ⮜

Another potential problem with some first-timers is that they may feel nothing at all when you first touch their clitoris. In this case, you want to play with your partner and tease her even more to get her to feel that first touch. Remember that your aim is to help your partner feel the very first stroke—to help her be instantly orgasmic—so play with her one stroke at a time before you increase the number of strokes and thereby extend the orgasm. At first it may take her a few strokes to get rolling, and once she does get rolling the sensations may only last for a short time.

You can practice giving your partner pleasure a single stroke at a time, or you can stroke your partner steadily till she starts noticeably feeling some pleasure. Then continue for however long the pleasure lasts, perhaps for only three or four more strokes. The goal here is for the pleasure giver to learn how to peak someone, and you obviously cannot do this by using only single strokes. Let your partner know what you are doing—that you want to get them to a place where they are having some contractions that you can notice, and then you will keep stroking until those contractions and sensations start to dissipate. When you stop and restart, the next peak will probably begin right away, or at least much quicker than the first one did.

The goal for the pleasure recipient is the same as always: to feel as much as they can with each stroke and with all the strokes combined. Each time you start a new peak there will be a first stroke, which the pleasure recipient can experience as an instant orgasm. The point here is that some flexibility in thinking is required to determine which approach will work best in each circumstance. You cannot rely on any specific formula, and learning from both possibilities—one stroke at a time as well as steady stroking—will yield benefits. Sometimes you can have a "one-stroke-at-a-time" session, and at other times you can dedicate the session to peaking by delivering more than one stroke at a time. You can even do both options in a single session. Some people are really good at feeling the first stroke yet have difficulty taking the intensity of the orgasm to a higher level. Others have challenges getting into the experience and feeling the pleasure right away, yet when they do get rolling the intensity easily magnifies. "Different strokes for different folks," as the saying goes. You have to pay attention to your partner and determine how to focus the game plan.

≳ Ways of Peaking ≶

There are different ways to peak someone. Any time you change your stroke you can usually expect a decrease in sensation, at least at first. There are exceptions to this rule. As we described in Chapter 6, some types of touch involve changing the stroke and moving all over the clitoris yet still allow you to continuously take your partner higher through your use of intention. Note that there is still a pattern involved with this kind of stroking. The pattern may be less obvious than delivering the same stroke repeatedly to the same spot, but it does exist. Usually, however, you will use your intention in synch with your change of stroke to deliberately bring your partner down. The change can be in the position of the stroke, the speed of the stroke, or the pressure of the stroke. The most typical way to bring someone down is to stop stroking altogether.

There are times when I'm giving pleasure to a trained woman when I peak her by barely skipping a beat. I stop stroking for a split second just to keep her attention, and then I begin with the same stroke again. She can use that tiny break to go down just a little, which will permit her to start flying higher right away when we start again. You can keep your partner going in this way for a long time, just skipping a beat every once in a while to prevent her attention from wandering. Of course, you can also take more time between strokes; that will depend on how you are feeling in response to her orgasm. The longer the break from stroking, the more the level of excitement will decrease. This is fine, as a trained woman can get back up very quickly, and she will enjoy a steeper climb when you do start stroking again.

When stroking a woman who is brand new to this kind of attention or early in her training, it usually is better to take a longer break, talk about what has just happened, and find out how she feels.

If one of you becomes thirsty, it is better to quench that thirst than to be thinking about being thirsty. We recommend speaking up if you want some water or other beverage, and keeping it handy so that you can stay in position while sipping. It is also okay to switch into a different position if either partner feels uncomfortable in any way. When a woman who is giving me pleasure stops to change positions, things always feel better when she restarts. The break is almost always justified and the pleasure increases. Sometimes people think they have to keep rubbing and rubbing without any breaks, but that is a recipe for trouble. For the sake of maintaining control of the session, it is also better for the pleasure giver to decide when to take the break rather than the pleasure recipient. A person cannot be at total effect (totally open to receiving pleasure) if they have to determine when to peak. Deciding to switch positions to one that's more comfortable could be the way a pleasure giver peaks his or her partner.

A fun way to peak almost any woman is to switch from a short stroke on her favorite clitoral spot to a long stroke down to her perineum and then up her introitus and inner labia. You can do this once, a couple of times, or even more. It will bring her down, but some women enjoy this attention even more than receiving fast strokes on their favored spot, especially women who are fairly new to this experience. She may prefer this slow, deliberate, long stroke to the shorter, faster one because she is more used to this kind of sensation and can associate pleasure with it more easily. Furthermore, you can use greater pressure when stroking places other than on the clitoris. This stroke also creates less performance anxiety for a woman who is still learning how to fully focus on each sensation. Remember that taking the arousal level down is not a bad thing; it is still part of the orgasm. There are two sides to any peak, and both sides of an orgasmic peak are places of pleasure. The down side is just a direction, and some people like it even better than going up. For example, when a man ejaculates, he is probably having his last peak, which means that most of those few seconds will be experienced while he's on his way down.

⇒ First-Stroke Mentality ⇐

After the break, whether it is for a few minutes or a split second, there will be a time to start stroking again (unless of course you've delivered the last peak). This is where the ability to get off on the first stroke will come in handy. The more the pleasure recipient can place their full attention on that initial touch, the quicker they can go higher and the more pleasure they will feel. Even if the break was a long one, being instantly orgasmic can allow a person to start feeling more pleasure right away after the break. During an extended orgasm many women, as well as some men, are able to experience pleasure and orgasmic sensation during the breaks, but at a somewhat reduced intensity.

You can tease your partner by telling her or him that this is the last peak, and then deliver another one. This may seem like it contradicts our advice to say what you are going to do and then to follow through. However, the goal here is to tease your partner into hopefully feeling more. You can say that you've changed your mind because they did so well, or that you are rewarding them with another peak. Then ask your partner to really feel the first stroke and to take it up in intensity with the next peak. At other times, of course, it is best to stick to your word and make that the final peak. In this way your partner will be unable to predict your next steps, which aids them in feeling more. You can ask your partner if she or he would like another peak. By looking at your lover's face and listening to the enthusiasm in her or his response, you can determine whether to give your partner another peak, to tease her or him some more, or to stop all together.

⇒ Between Peaks ⇐

During the break, depending on how long it is, each partner has a choice about where to focus their attention. The pleasure recipient can continue to feel as much as possible by keeping their attention on their genitals. She or he can sort of catch her or his breath and get ready to feel more soon. Both partners can discuss the previous peak and acknowledge how pleasurable it was and still is. The pleasure giver can coach the other partner by reminding him or her to relax, by describing how the next peak is going to go even higher, or by telling them how you want them to focus their attention on the first stroke and on each stroke that follows. The pleasure recipient can ask for a specific type of stroke, if desired. You can shift positions and quench your thirst if necessary.

➤ Peaking by Changing the Stroke ≼

Remember that changing the nature of the stroke in any way will usually result in a peak. During a session, you can alternate between cycles in which you use slow strokes and cycles in which you use quicker ones. As you continue alternating, notice how your partner responds, and tell them what you notice. You can also alternate between lighter and firmer pressures with each cycle. You can vary the length of the peaks, stroking lightly for a good number of strokes, then stroking more firmly a very few times, and so on. You can also mix up hard-stroke and slow-stroke cycles with fast-stroke and light-stroke cycles. The possibilities are nearly endless.

We want to reemphasize the importance of the pleasure giver's intention in creating heightened sensation in his or her partner. This means that the stroke itself is less important than what your intention is when giving it. The same stroke with different intentions can be used to take someone higher or to bring them down. Usually light and fast strokes increase tumescence, and hard and slow strokes decrease tumescence, but with the proper intention one can use any stroke to go in either direction. Sometimes you can even use a specific stroke to bring your partner down quite a bit. The right combination of your intention, a firmer and slower stroke (usually), and perhaps moving off the spot can take your partner down. Sometimes when Vera and I are doing demonstrations, her arousal level gets so high that the spectators are unable to keep up. By deliberately bringing Vera down a little, I can help the spectators notice and learn more.

➤ Peaking and Control ≼

As we have repeatedly stated, to experience the most pleasure a person must surrender her or his nervous system into someone else's care. To make this happen the pleasure giver must manifest control over the partner's tumescence. By peaking someone at the right time you demonstrate that control. Control is really about doing what the other person wants, and doing it even before they may realize they want it. We're not talking about forcing someone to do things they don't want to do. It is more about noticing the other person's frame of mind, getting into agreement with where they are, and staying one step ahead of them when possible.

This is where peaking is so important. If one were to keep stroking beyond the point where the pleasure is rising to the point where it is actually falling, then the pleasure recipient will not feel taken care of and will balk at surrendering. By stopping on the dime, by paying close attention and noticing when it is a good time for a break, you stay in the driver's seat and increase your control. Imagine dancing with your partner. You want to make it fun for both of you, so you swing your partner around and around, yet if you keep doing that same movement both of you will probably get dizzy and your partner will start wondering when you are going to stop twirling her. However, if you twirl your partner a couple of times, catch her, do some two-stepping together, and then twirl her again in a slightly different pattern, you will keep your partner interested. Your partner will look forward to getting twirled instead of dreading it.

⋗ Know When to Break the Rules ⋖

We have stressed how it is better to peak your partner too soon than too late. That is a good rule of thumb, but like any rule it can be overdone, because it is equally true that people like a consistent, dependable stroke that increases their pleasure with each stroke. To repeatedly peak your partner too early could put a damper on the possibility of more sensation. It is of utmost importance to pay close attention to your partner and to notice whether they are still appreciating your continued, reliable stroking, and to keep delivering that stroke for as long as you can. The closer you can get to the point of diminishing returns, the higher you will be able to take your partner. This is where experience and practice will make you a better judge of exactly when to peak someone.

A pleasure giver has to learn to trust his or her own feelings. Whether the feelings emanate from your gut, your genitals, or your brain, know that you should follow them. Notice that we listed the brain last. That's because when you start thinking too much while you are pleasuring someone, your attention has already wandered away from their pleasure and your pleasure. You must remain aware of your gut feelings, which are evidenced by your mind realizing whether it is time for a break or time to continue stroking. As we've stated, if you are unsure, or if you are questioning whether or not to peak your partner, then it is a good time to do so or at least to tell them that you might. Words are very powerful, and the precise communication of a gut feeling will more often than not get your partner back on track. By talking through what you are feeling you remain in control, and you allow your partner to thoroughly surrender.

⟫ Training Peaks ⟪

Early in your training with your partner, you may ask your partner to let you know when to peak them, when you have gone too long, and how they wish to be peaked. If you are the one being pleasured, before your partner even starts touching you, you can let him or her know that you will be offering suggestions about when to take a break, for how long, and what change of stroke you prefer. Remember to give lots of acknowledgments along with your instructions and suggestions. The more appreciation you verbalize, the easier it will be to give an instruction that your partner will gladly fulfill. Just say, "I'd love a break" or "This is a perfect point to peak me." Earlier in the chapter we described how it is far more fun to have someone peak you than to tell them when to do so. When you are training someone to learn when and how to peak, you will usually have to take a more responsible role and coach them till they get it. After a while you can tell your partner that they are to trust their own intuition and peak you as they see fit. Tell them you will give them feedback about how well they are doing. At any time, you can still request whatever you desire, including when to peak you.

These peaking suggestions are valid for pleasuring men and women. It is especially tricky for men to learn to pleasure women, as touching a clitoris precisely is more difficult than touching a penis. To complicate matters, mastering the timing of peaking is not easy at first. This is why it is so important for women to know their own bodies and be able to communicate to their partners exactly how they want to be touched and how to peak them appropriately.

⋙ Peaking Before Ejaculation ⋘

Although penises are easily located and usually quite simple to manipulate and to pleasure, they can present a challenge regarding when, how, and how often to peak a man who is about to ejaculate. For a man, there is a point of no return, and peaking him at the right moment before this occurs can add to his pleasure. Each man is different with regard to what it takes to make him ejaculate and what it takes to keep him from ejaculating. Some men have trained themselves to hold off from ejaculating through Tantric practices or other means. Some men are either so sensitive or perhaps so horny that just a little stimulation will trigger them to start squirting. Most men lie somewhere in between. To enjoy the most pleasure possible, a man, like a woman, has to surrender his nervous system and go for as much sensation as he can so that his partner can take full control of his arousal. He must train his partner about when to peak him at the right moment in order to extend his pleasure. Once she gets the timing down, she will be able to pleasure him much more than he ever realized was possible.

One of the signs of a man's imminent ejaculation is a secondary erection, in which the head of his penis becomes more bulbous and turns a purplish color.

There are a number of ways to peak a man; that is, to stop him from ejaculating. The easiest and perhaps the best way is to stop stimulating him close to but before his imminent release. Just take your hand off of his penis for a short time. Then when you start stroking again you can take him even higher with the next peak, which may be quite short, as his level of arousal may not have dropped very far. A few strokes may bring him back up to where he was or even higher. The longer you wait between peaks the farther down he will go, yet the next ride up may still be quite quick in comparison to the earlier one.

A second way to peak a man is to squeeze the head of his penis in your hand—firmly but not too tightly, and without using any up-and-down or side-to-side movement. This action will usually bring him down, though some men like it so much that they will ejaculate. You have to experiment with the right pressure and communicate with your partner to find out what pressure and timing work best. Don't feel bad if you mistime a peak and he either squirts (because you were too late) or did not get high enough (because you were too early with your stopping and squeezing).

A third way to peak a man is to press his ejaculatory duct through his perineum using two or three fingers. Firm pressure is required, and you will only have to press for a second or two. Do not press so hard that it hurts, just enough to stop the urge to ejaculate from continuing.

We suggest that you talk to your partner before and during the act, and then when he is close to squirting he can let you know. He can say, "I'm getting really excited now" or "I will ejaculate in a few strokes" or "I'm really close" or simply "Please stop." Then he can let you know when he has calmed down enough for you to begin again.

You will have to choose, or he can recommend, the best technique to use to peak him. While you are learning, you can ask him, "How close are you to ejaculating?" After a while you will become familiar with his bodily responses and pretty much know where he is. At some point he may ask you to stop. If you want to ejaculate him, you can respond with, "That's nice, but I'm taking you all the way this time." You can also keep peaking him even if he is asking for you to ejaculate him; let him know that you are in control and will squirt him on your own timetable. You will learn how long to wait between peaks, that is, when to start stroking again. You can deliberately restart quickly after a very short break, knowing in advance that it may only take a couple of strokes to get him back to the point of no return. Play with that edge for a few peaks, stop briefly, deliver a couple more strokes, and so on. Most guys really enjoy this technique.

You can peak a man anytime—even if he is not on the edge of ejaculation—because you want to take a break, in order to readjust your hands or body, or, very importantly, when his attention is about to wander or is already wandering. Peaking him will keep you in control of his nervous system, allowing you to take him to a higher place than he would otherwise go. Other excellent reasons to take a break are to move stray pubic hairs out of the way or to apply more lubricant. Tell him what you are up to so that there are no surprises and he can surrender to you fully without wondering what you are doing. Good communication is just as important when pleasuring a man as it is when pleasuring a woman.

⋙ Go Peak Yourself ⋘

The more thoroughly you understand the intricate nature of your own body's ability to use peaking to increase your level of tumescence, and the more effectively you can communicate this to your partner, the better your orgasms will be. For this reason it is important to practice peaking your own body, whether you are a man or a woman. It is fun to do, allows for more intense sensation, and gives you skills to apply with your partner as both pleasure giver and pleasure recipient.

Most men—and many women, too—masturbate just to relieve tension. With the peaking exercise we deliberately build as much tension as we can before releasing it. Every time we stop and start again we increase the amount of intensity we can feel. I remember when I tried peaking myself after having taken my first sensuality class. Using a *Playboy* magazine calendar, I peaked myself to each girl of the month, and then when I decided to ejaculate I went back to my favorite photo to finish myself off. I came close to ejaculating with each fantasy girl and stopped myself either by removing my hand for a few seconds (I had to turn the page) or by pressing my ejaculatory duct through my perineum and then removing my hand for a few seconds (see Figure 24 on the next page).

Most women do not have to worry about ejaculating (some women can ejaculate, of course, but this will not necessarily signal the end of their orgasm). As long as they relax their bodies, they can continue stimulating themselves to whatever level of arousal they can attain before their mind starts to wander and the intensity decreases. Practice on yourself by experimenting with all the different ways of peaking that we have described in this chapter. Find out which methods you like best, how long you like to wait between

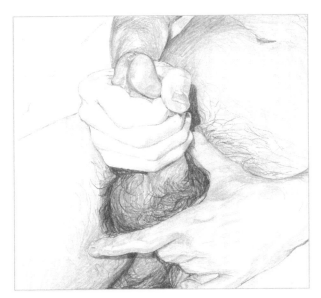

Figure 24.
Pressure on
perineum to
prevent ejaculation

peaks, and what you like to do between peaks. Be ready to feel that next first stroke. By practicing and observing how your body works, specifically with regard to peaking, you will gain an immense amount of knowledge that you can pass on to your partner.

In order to become the best possible giver of pleasure, you will have to incorporate the art of peaking into your practice until it becomes second nature. It is all about your ability to stay focused and keep your attention on the pleasure that is occurring in your partner. You must be able to pick up on slight changes that signify a potential retreat, and then beat your partner to the punch by pulling the proverbial rug out from under them. Becoming proficient at peaking is often one of the last and most challenging parts of becoming a great lover. The information in this chapter, practiced regularly, gives you a good foundation for becoming just that.

CHAPTER 8

Closing Words

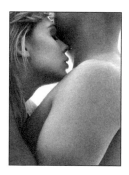

*W*e have given you quite a bit of information in these pages. It will take some time for you to digest everything, put it all together, and come out as one of the best sexers in the world. You will have to do the work, practice what you have learned, and apply as much of the information as is feasible. Pursuing this knowledge has consumed (naturally very pleasurably) a good part of Vera's and my life. This is the fourth book we have written on the subject of pleasure and orgasm, and each time we learn more. The information in our books, especially this one, is a culmination of all we have discovered. Our students and workshop attendees have cumulatively paid thousands of dollars to learn what we have imparted here for just the price of this book. You may learn more quickly if you were to come study with us, but with dedicated application of what you have read here, you can become a great sexer and sensualist.

A person could also use this information to start their own sensual-teaching practice. We are available for consultation to anyone who wishes to begin a business in sensual pleasure. There are very few places in the world where one can find appropriate facilitators for this kind of pleasure, especially women's pleasure. We only know of teachers in California, New York City, and Hawaii. We would love for more people to have "hands-on" access to these techniques. A huge opportunity exists for those who are interested in making pleasure a priority and who wish to create a business from this work.

The title of our first book, *Extended Massive Orgasm,* appealed to some people and created apprehension in others. We even received e-mails from a few feminist groups who, without having read our books, thought that we were placing performance pressure on women who had trouble reaching orgasm. We apologize to these women because our intention was to create an easier and more gratifying way for women to experience pleasure. Our books are really all about that. Perhaps the name of the book seemed to promise too much, yet we are glad we were able to reach those who wanted to take their sensual lives to the next level. Hopefully the title of this book will have a different effect and will attract women who believe they can learn to feel more sensual pleasure. We also want to attract readers whose orgasms are already wonderful but who want to take things even higher. We think we have accomplished both.

⇒ Choose Pleasure ⇐

We want to touch once more on the importance of attitude in the creation of pleasure for yourself and your partner. One of the least hedonistic or sensual places in which to dwell is scarcity (Scare City). If you see signs pointing to Scare City, go in the opposite direction. In this mental place, opportunities and experiences that could be seen as gratifying and fun instead appear torturous and frightening.

How can we get from scarcity to feeling more abundant and feeling good about ourselves? The answer lies in one's attitude, in one's appreciation of the small things that are constantly happening to us and around us. It is about being more conscious, being aware, and focusing your attention on the present moment. It is about looking through the proverbial rose-colored glasses and seeing the proverbial glass as half full or more. It is about recognizing your surplus and giving it away. These all sound like the same attributes that we describe in creating and experiencing IOs and EMOs. There is no coincidence here. In order to create pleasure, and in order to feel abundance and gratitude, a person must devote himself or herself to a mindset that will promote these qualities.

When we are focused on the future (what we will get or not get) or the past (what we have lacked or lost), we fall into that place of scarcity. The same goes for orgasm. We have to remain in present time and we have to appreciate what's happening now to shift into extended pleasure. All it takes is switching one's mindset, yet where is that switch, and how do we flip it?

It all goes back to embracing the viewpoint that the world is perfect the way it is. This perfection includes good, bad, and ugly. It involves seeing things as they are, not as you think they should be—as in some kind of utopia or some future heaven that awaits you. It is about right now, about what is. It is playing the cards that we are dealt and judging them to be the right cards no matter what. There is no throwing in the cards for new cards until you play your hand the way it was dealt. The only thing you can change is your attitude. When you change your attitude you can see things from a new perspective. From wherever you are, there are always ways to lose and there are always ways to win.

Sexually speaking, the same is true. The pleasure is in you, not in who is doing it to you. Most people decide whether someone is good-looking and then assume that being touched by that attractive person would be wonderful. Or they assume that being touched by someone who looks "ugly" would be less exciting. We as human beings have the ability to get off fantastically no matter who is touching us, ourselves included. When we are out of agreement with things—when we judge the situation or our partner to be wrong—we limit ourselves with regard to the pleasure available. This is due to living in some other moment besides the present moment, either the past or the future. The ability to feel pleasure with any kind of touch comes with training and with the capacity to see the perfection in every circumstance.

This ability to be utterly in the "now" is the defining characteristic of sensuality. We all have this potential. As we described in the Introduction, throughout this book we have kept you in a perpetual state of arousal. We have practically left out any discussion of coming down. We purposely wanted you to stay focused on the pleasure of the first stroke and to continue receiving every stroke as if it were the only one. This is what we mean when we talk about being sensual: to feel every stroke and to be present to all of your pleasure potential.

A journey begins with the first step. We see lots of journeys in your future. If you wish to reach us in between any of your journeys, feel free to e-mail us at verasteve@aol.com.

Frequently Asked Questions

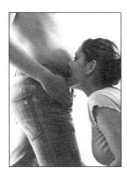

We receive e-mails from all over the world, yet the questions posed in them are often very similar. The best kind of question to ask is one that reveals something about you and that feels risky to ask. Simply by asking questions you will open new doors to creating more pleasure. The root of the word itself comes from the Latin word *questare,* which is also the root for the word "quest." Here are a few quests we have gone on with our readers in the past couple of years.

 I am attached to the idea of "loving" the man I surrender to, but I fear I create a kind of catch-22 for myself. I fall in love very, very rarely and thus enter long periods of sexual aloneness. I desire to have many satisfying sensual and sexual experiences, but that is so difficult when I have to feel a lot of emotional attachment in order to surrender.

Can you advise me of any concrete (baby) steps that I could take to make my life more fun and satisfying until my legendary love appears?

— *Baby Steps*

Dear Baby Steps,
Remember that you are not surrendering to any individual; you
are surrendering to your own pleasure. That means if you let some
man take control of your nervous system, he is not defeating you; he is serving you.

We believe that we are all responsible for our lives and that we pick and
choose according to our greatest desires. You have to decide what your priority is: pleasure or waiting for Prince Charming. Meanwhile, we suggest that
you practice pleasuring yourself with your own hand or with a water hose;
you can find appropriate exercises in this book.

Vera and I started out as research partners. She was married, and I was in
love with another woman. We created great pleasure together without a whole
lot of emotional attachment, and then we began to fall in love with each other,
slowly yet continuously. Today we have one of the best relationships we know
of. Deciding what to do is up to you. It is okay to wait for the right guy, but from
your question we wonder if you may want to go more in the other direction.

 Until last year, I had a very healthy libido, having experienced
many years of enjoyable sexual encounters. Oddly, since getting
married and having a baby, *nothing* turns me on any longer. I realize a woman's libido can be reduced after childbirth (and I do still breast-feed),
but it's been seventeen months and I have absolutely no interest in sex of any
kind.

You say two of the biggest enemies of turn-on are anger and doubt. I don't
feel particularly "angry," though I've always wished my husband had a higher
sex drive and was more demonstrative. I've considered "doubt," but all I can
come up with is the fact that I might be a little detached from my pussy since
childbirth. My son weighed nine pounds and I had lots of stitches. Not that
I'm afraid sex will hurt (we've done it; it doesn't). It's more of an awareness that
my body has changed slightly.

I do get a reasonable amount of sleep, for a mom. I'm not overly stressed
and I like the way my body looks. I just started reading *To Bed or Not to Bed*

and I made an appointment for a blood test, just in case. Overall, I love my life. In many ways I've never been happier, but I know that I'm not being true to myself by living without sex and being so out of touch with my sensuality.

— _Libidoless Mom_

 Dear Libidoless Mom,

We have met many women who have refrained from sex after birthing, often for as long as two years. If you want to have more sensuality in your life you will have to be more deliberate. People find lots of reasons _not_ to have sensual experiences. You will have to look a little harder and deeper to find reasons to have them. We call these things "assigned authors," and they can come in the form of a friend, a book, a course, or whatever excuse you can use. People (women) do not have to feel in heat or totally aroused in order to have a pleasure experience. They do have to admit that they feel kind of flat sexually yet would like to go for it anyway. Once you start, the juices will flow and you will have fun no matter how little you felt like it at first. On the other hand, you do not have to have sex; it is not necessary to life, like breathing and eating. By just asking this question you are on the path to more pleasure.

By the way, from your letter and knowing what we know about women, we would say that you do have anger toward your husband. You do not have to. Choose pleasure. Talk to your husband nicely (use the training cycle) about making more offers to you, and be receptive in your responses to them.

 Thanks so much for your elegant response. I would love to have a bit more clarity, if I may. I understand the "assigned authors" to be things/people I can use to stimulate my interest in sex. Is this correct? How would this work?

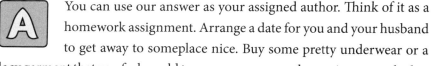 You can use our answer as your assigned author. Think of it as a homework assignment. Arrange a date for you and your husband to get away to someplace nice. Buy some pretty underwear or a lacy garment that you feel would turn your guy on, and more importantly that turns you on. Create a little basket of goodies, such as chocolate or berries or

whatever both of you like to taste, and include something to drink. Make sure you have some music, flowers, and the like—items to stimulate all five of your senses. Imagine a fantasy that you can use to turn each other on. Create the space, arrange the time, and handle all his resistances, because there surely will be some. We recommend reading about how to create an all-day pleasure experience in our book *Extended Massive Orgasm*. Although it is designed for pleasuring a woman, you can use it to inspire ideas about how to pleasure a guy, too. Give him the most erotic, fun time he has ever had.

In addition, we also want you to get off in whatever way you want to at least once a day. These are your assignments, and we are your assigned authors. If you do not follow our instructions, it means you are not giving us enough power and we will have to charge you. Does this make it clearer?

 My issues surrounding sexual encounters center on one thing: I have herpes and feel like I have a scarlet "H" blazoned across my chest. When I am in a relationship I feel I am held back sexually because of my diagnosis. I believe I need to be honest about it, but I also worry that it makes the man not want me. I feel tarnished and ashamed and like I can't have a full sex life. I don't know exactly how to talk to a man about this issue. I have not had a breakout in at least five years, but it feels like a weight that holds me down. My biggest fear is that no one will want me. It has taken so much for me to ask this question, and I so appreciate your help.

— *Scarlet H*

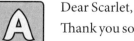 Dear Scarlet,

Thank you so much for asking such a gutsy question. Many people have herpes; some people have it without even knowing they do. When you meet the right guy, telling him you have herpes won't prevent him from loving you. Although herpes is not a minor issue, you are the one who is making it into a big one. You are the one who is using it to prevent you from enjoying further intimacy. Yes, you will have to discuss it with anyone whom you become interested in, though your diagnosis does not have to be given out with your name and phone number to each guy you meet. You can wait until you know the person better and are sure of how intimate you would like to become with him.

I am sure there are herpes support groups in most cities and definitely on the Internet. You may even meet some guy who is in the same boat as you. There are many more difficult issues that people face about intimacy and relationships. You do not have to be ashamed of having herpes, as it is so common. You have not had any outbreaks in a while, and from what I've read it is fairly safe to engage in sexual activity when the patient isn't having an outbreak. And, of course, you can have your partner wear a condom for further protection. As you know, we teach manual stimulation, which is the best way to produce pleasure in both men and women. When a person washes with soap and water after a sensual session in which only manual stimulation occurs, there will be no spreading of the herpes virus (providing there are no open cuts on the pleasure giver's hands). Another safeguard is for the pleasure giver to wear latex gloves, in which case it is necessary to use a water-soluble lubricant. We have never seen a herpes blister on the clitoris itself. It is made of a very strong tissue and rarely gets any diseases, and its only function is pleasure. So put your attention on your clitoris and your pleasure instead of on a virus.

My husband and I are just beginning to venture into sexual relations after an extended break. I made the decision to suspend sex to make sure we are both radiantly happy no matter what. He is not aggressive in lovemaking, although when we met he was more so. I decided to explore the realm of submissive/dominant and began to take the dominant role, and to my curiosity and delight he responded well in so many ways: emotionally, sexually, lovingly. It took nerve for me to do that, but it is my main interest to make sure that we and our energies harmonize.

My question is this: As the dominant, I am on top, which keeps me from being as relaxed as I would be if I were underneath, receiving. When he is eating my pussy, I am straddling him. What might you suggest in terms of my being able to relax my body and my pussy?

— *Not Quite Dominatrix*

 Dear Not Quite,

Thank you for exposing so much of yourself in your question. The more a person is willing to reveal about themselves under the right circumstances, especially when it is scary to do so, the more they are likely to reap special benefits that they did not even see coming.

Role playing can be fun, and one can play many roles. You and your husband can try different roles and positions. You are not stuck with one role for life and neither is he. It is more difficult to relax when straddling than when lying down, so find some pillows that could add support and make it easier for you to relax while straddling. You can also use your imagination. If you are playing the dominant role, dominate your husband so that he sucks you off or stimulates you with his hands while you are in a more relaxed position, like on your back. In other words, if you are giving him orders, then order him to behave the way you want him to. Who's in charge here? Communicate your desires to your husband, and it sounds as though he will come through like a champ. Your true desires will be fulfilled. Show him our DVD of Vera lying on her back being stimulated manually for an hour.

 1. I'm pretty certain that I am experiencing EMOs (I haven't yet read your books, so I am going on other women's descriptions). What I find is that my orgasms can go on and on, but I don't necessarily ever feel "done." I usually stop at a random point, or when my partner is done. My question is, how do you get a feeling of being complete, if there is such a thing? I hope you understand what I mean. Because it seems as though you can continue "riding the waves" forever.

2. Sometimes I get the feeling that my husband thinks my orgasmic-ness and desire are overwhelming. I get orgasmic almost immediately and I could go on and on. But I feel like I am a burden to him. He only likes to come once.

That's usually when I "finish" also, because I love the after-cuddling, but then I would like to continue. Sometimes we do. I don't quite understand this dynamic and it's uncomfortable. I feel so happy with my evolving sexuality and sensuality and I don't want to feel like I'm being "too much" or a burden to my man.

3. I'd love some ideas on introducing more sensuality to my husband. He doesn't particularly enjoy it or have any interest in learning about it. He likes to do anything involving my pussy or breasts or intercourse, but he doesn't enjoy his own skin being caressed, and he isn't really into kissing much, either. I feel stumped by all this. I love going slowly and building and teasing and kissing, and I really miss that.

4. Steve, when you signed my book you wrote, "Take no prisoners." What does that mean? I've been smiling about it since.

— *Feeling Kinda Exposed*

 Dear Exposed,

1. When we describe EMOs we are specifically talking about manual to clitoral stimulation. You can experience EMOs in other ways, too; they're just less intense. You write that you are done when your husband is done, which sounds to us like you are describing intercourse. When I stimulate Vera's clitoris, we can do it for five minutes or fifteen minutes or an hour or whatever we feel like. There is no specific end point, no proclamation saying "The End." She is off to the races on the first stroke, and the intensity is very strong compared to a tensed-up crotch sneeze, which usually lasts for ten seconds. Hers keeps going and going, with peaks, of course. As long as she remains relaxed, her whole body is in orgasm.

Often after bringing her up for however long I desire, I will use intention combined with a change in the pressure of my touch to indicate when we are "finished." This brings her level of excitement down a few notches, as we describe in our books. We also use intercourse as a way of coming down. This coming down is very pleasurable and is part of the orgasm; she is still contracting and feeling intense sensation as the orgasm slowly recedes. It is a way to complete the sexual cycle; however, sometimes we forgo the down ride and let her stay at a high level of tumescence. This can feel uncomfortable to some women at first, but after a number of times most learn to enjoy the feeling. We do not suggest trying to function or drive a car in this state.

It would be best to have your husband learn to control your level of tumescence—that is, learn how to bring you up and how to take you down. You are not insatiable; you just require lots of attention. Once he learns his craft he will be able to take you higher for longer, and you will be gratified.

2. Again, it seems you are describing intercourse. Have your husband learn to pleasure you manually, which he can do for however long you like. He will not feel overwhelmed. His finger will not lose its erection. Then when you want to, you can pleasure him at the end with intercourse or however you choose, and then cuddle. I like to give Vera a long orgasm and sometimes we only do that; at other times she wants to give me orgasmic pleasure, too, with hands, legs, mouth, or pussy. Once I have ejaculated, I do not want to start stimulating her again. She can stimulate me to where I am close to ejaculating but do not go over, and then I can keep going and stimulate her some more if she so desires. When your husband can learn to pleasure you without "Mr. Happy" having to stay erect for the entire happy hour, he will not feel burdened. He will feel like a hero.

3. Above all, guys like to succeed. They love to win. You have to train your husband, and the best way to train is with lots of rewards, lots of wins. Then he will do whatever you want. Do not ask for the sky and the moon all at once. Ask for little things and appreciate those, and slowly and sensually you will build him into the exact man you are manifesting. When he does kiss you, tell him how good that makes you feel without creating any pressure for him to have to do more. You say you like to go slowly, so here is your chance. Enjoy his resistances; your pussy power is way too strong, when properly used, for him to succeed at resisting for long. Learn to communicate with him on a more intimate level, which you do by telling the truth in a kind way, not with anger. Put your attention on pleasure, not on your doubts, and definitely not on your "righteous" anger. Manipulation, when used for everyone's fun, is not a bad thing.

4. "Take no prisoners" is a metaphor for making sure you fulfill your erotic desires by killing all your enemies like anger and doubt. It's like saying "Go for

the gold." I may have been wrong: There is one prisoner you get to keep (if you get my drift in the context of my answer to the last question), so make sure it is more like summer camp than a concentration camp.

Thanks for the great questions. They were fun to answer. You definitely have some wonderful appetite.

 Can you describe a good way that I can give my boyfriend a really gratifying ejaculation with my hands?

— *Raggedy Handy*

 Dear Raggedy,

We love this question because we have noticed that many women can get a guy off without any problem, except they kind of space out when he starts to squirt. We included some information on this topic in Chapter 7 of this book ("The Pleasure of Peaking"), and we just want to remind you that when you are ready to squirt him, keep feeling your own pleasure and keep communicating with him. Let him know that you are ready to squirt him or make him come or whatever words you like. I remember one woman who said to me, "I am no longer fooling around; this time I'm taking you all the way."

A good stroke to use is to place one hand fully around his penis, milking it all the way from bottom to top using whatever speed he likes. Although the emphasis is on the upstroke, do not remove your hand when going back down to the base of his penis but feel his penis all the way down, too. You can use your second hand to stimulate his engorged "hidden" cock by stroking your fingertips along his perineum, under his scrotum, again placing the emphasis on the upstroke, moving in the direction from anus to scrotum. This stroke can synchronize with the one on his penis—that is, both hands stroking upward at the same time and at a similar speed. I like fairly light pressure on my penis and a little more pressure on my perineum area. You will have to find out from your partner what amount of pressure he prefers.

Besides this stroke, you can use almost any pleasurable stroke on his penis, a long or short stroke, with one hand or two. Once you've established a good stroke, don't peak him here by changing the stroke; perhaps use more intention and maybe a little more speed as you approach the point of no return. As he starts to ejaculate please do not stop stroking him, which we have noticed that some women do; maintain as much contact between your hand and his penis as you can. If anything, increase your attention on the pleasure in your hands as he begins to ejaculate. You can let him know, "Here it comes; big gobs of ejaculate landed on your belly" (or the ceiling). Keep doing the same stroke for the first few explosions. After the early bursts continue with the same motion, lightening up and slowing down a little with each stroke. Keep doing this as long as he has sensation and is being pleasured. This can last for quite a few strokes as long as you keep reducing the pressure. Then you can wipe him off by lightly dabbing the towel against his penis without including any rubbing or friction.

My brain's libido is stuck desiring a man who has no desire for me. Currently I have resigned myself to remaining friends with him rather than continuing to be occasional lovers. My body and soul loved having sex with him. I love his smell, his sweat; his vibe sends me into sublime revelry. I am so turned on when I walk five steps into his apartment that I can barely contain myself. But he is currently involved with someone else, and I need to move on.

I have had other men since him, but my brain lingers on thoughts that compare these lovers to him. So far, other men smell sour or not right, the vibe is not there, and sometimes certain parts of them make me absolutely gag. When I was with him I loved being covered with his sweat and his being. I haven't seen him in nearly a year, but I just can't move on. Trying to find someone to re-create those feelings with has been so difficult, yet I am trying super hard to have an open mind. When he pops into my brain (which seems to be every day), I even whisper a mantra to myself to get him out of my head: "He has no love for me, and this is not working well."

I have been doing my best with self-pleasuring, but after months and months I still feel that I am not moving forward. I am ever so tired of this one-sided love affair.

— Ms. Victim

Dear Ms. Victim,

Poor baby, such a victim! Unfortunately your plight is apparently shared by a number of women, some of whom call themselves Goddesses. We feel conflicted responses, such as wanting to hug you and put your head in our lap and say, "There, there," but also wanting to smack you and say, "Wake up and live." But you are living and you're making the choice to lose, yet you are looking for help, which is a good sign.

The past is the past, and it is time to move on, as you say. First of all, do not go out anymore with anyone who smells sour. Next, you can do a spring cleaning on the old guy to remove all that charge. (Read Chapter 4 in our book *To Bed or Not to Bed* for this and other exercises.) Finally, do a better job on your self-pleasuring, which means placing more emphasis on setting up your space. Create a worthy environment in which to cherish yourself and fall in love with yourself by doing the mirror exercise with unabashed lustful love for yourself and your exquisite body. The more love you heap upon yourself, the less neediness you will project and the better the guy you will attract.

You are responsible for your life, and everything that has led you up to this moment was perfect just the way it was. You are now ready for the best time of your life. Take the bull by the horns; take the tiger by the tail. Come out to California and learn what orgasm is really about. Take enjoyment from whatever you do, including thinking about your past. It is your destiny! It's up to you.

I have done some meditating and visualizing, and I hear and see desirable outcomes to my situations. These serve as crystal-clear confirmation that what I desire is coming to me, particularly when I'm not looking for it. (I'll be visualizing about furniture or career, and a great guy will show up, unbidden.) I also have a level of intuitive knowledge that I am beginning to learn to listen to, but occasionally I'm very quick to draw conclusions about how to get there. I lunge at what I see coming to me (because I can see it), and I suspect I get in the way of its arrival.

What I have difficulty with is my ego surrendering the "how" to allow for greater co-creation. I'm an electrical engineer, and I'm often a creator all by myself. I feel like I'm getting in the way of the universe delivering my desires to me, because I keep peeking in the oven to look at the soufflé.

— Confused

 Dear Confused,

This sounds a lot like psycho-babble, yet we see a real question hidden here. Yes, your doubt will clog up the works and slow the delivery. In your case, it sounds as though doubt and uncertainty are showing up in the form of impatience. It's like you're planting a seed and then digging it up every day to check on its progress.

You have to get your desires straight, prioritized, and pleasure-oriented, and you must appreciate any movement toward your goals. The soufflé comment is a cute analogy. It's okay to look in the oven; maybe get a glass window so you don't have to open the oven door. And don't forget to enjoy the aroma as the soufflé is baking. Feel your mouth moisten and salivating as it anticipates a great feast. It's all in the attitude.

 It has been a very long time since I have been in an open sexual arena. I've been divorced for two years, and I've had no sex for the last five years. I have had a close male friend for seven years. I don't know how to make the jump into letting him know of my passionate desires for him. I feel like I am fourteen, with the blazing appetite of a fifty-year-old woman. How do I switch gears with him without coming on too strong? There is a tremendous static in the air—like a crackling energy. What do I say? What do I do? I know that I am on the cusp of something really big.

— Fallen

Dear Fallen,

Ain't love great? Being that you are fifty and not fourteen, you can communicate your feelings to this man without worrying what the heck the rest of the world thinks. The meek and timid may inherit the earth, but do you have time to wait? We do not know his story—is he married, divorced, what? And we do not know what his feelings are for you. He may have the same feelings for you as you do for him, and he may have his own reasons for not talking about them to you. On the other hand, maybe he just wants to be friends and does not have the same feelings. You have to find out.

You can ask him directly how he feels toward you. You can slowly tell him of your passionate feelings, being alert to his responses, so that if he shows any resistance you can play with it. You know, use the old push-pull game. You can let loose your feminine charms and your turn-on and play with his male response. What man would not want to hear that some Goddess is hot for him? You can seduce him if he is reluctant but shows some interest in you. You can talk to his friends about him to find out more. You can ask him out on a date, maybe a walk in the park, and get to know him even better. Read our book *To Bed or Not to Bed* for more hints on how to seduce this lucky guy. The worst that can happen is that you strike out with him, but if you don't take some swings you will never know. Go for the fun.

 I'm a little confused by your discussion of female orgasm. I didn't learn how to have an orgasm from a man. I learned it from self-pleasuring on my own as a preteen and teenager. My orgasms, both by myself and with a man, do sometimes have the build-up and then release—what you describe as a "crotch sneeze"—and sometimes I suppose I am tensing up as I move toward them. But I didn't learn that from anyone, just from my own body. My orgasms are quite pleasurable, and I sort of enjoy the intensity of the build-up and release, especially with a partner.

I have always been able to have orgasms during intercourse, and I love them. I suspect that I naturally created some of the connections you describe in your books, because I don't think my clitoris is particularly close to my vagina. In addition, I have noticed that manual and/or oral stimulation before and during intercourse make a difference for me.

Of course, I am definitely intrigued by the idea of having the feelings of pleasure go on longer than they do, as in an EMO, and I can completely understand that if a woman felt pressured to come the way that her male partner does it could be problematic, so I commend you for setting things straight. But my question is: Do I need to change the way I do things? Am I missing out on something? Is there something wrong with crotch sneezes?

I really enjoy the feeling of connection that I experience with a partner during intercourse, and though I certainly feel connected during other types of stimulation it's not the same feeling. Is this normal? Is it okay to enjoy intercourse as much as, and possibly more than, manual stimulation?

Basically, I feel in agreement with my own sexuality, and I don't think there's anything wrong with me, but after reading your books it appears that there's another perspective and experience out there that I wasn't aware of.

— *Crotch Sneezeophiliac*

Dear Sneezeophiliac,

You are in a very good place. You have orgasms and you can have them with intercourse. The only trouble with being in a good place is that it is difficult to get to a better one from there, as you do not have the bad chasing your ass down the block. Dealing with getting from good to better is our forte, so we appreciate your question.

First of all, we do not do amputations, so you get to keep everything you already have, including your "crotch sneezes." We *do* offer women a way to have a different, and we think important, new perspective about what is possible in the arena of orgasmic potential. This will not require that you give anything up, but rather that you include a new discipline or practice that takes time and attention, hopefully of the fun variety, as you explore your body's ability to feel. You can practice on your own, practice with your partner, or for the quickest results practice with us (pricier than the first two options).

There are plenty of women who love to have intercourse—maybe not as many as truth will tell, but still plenty, and our work only enhances this ability. At this time, you may enjoy intercourse more than manual stimulation. There are intimacy and conditioning factors that prejudice many people toward intercourse, and, again, we do not want you to give it up. We would, however, remind you that you have not yet enjoyed great manual stimulation, so you can hardly compare the two at this point in your life. This may turn out to be a great competition, with you as the direct beneficiary!

 I have been wavering back and forth between going cold turkey from vibrator to manual, but I can't seem to bring myself to cut the cord. I have had a plug-in for twelve years that gives me orgasms galore. Yet I have had an orgasm only once while being stimulated manually by a guy. At age thirty-three, I feel quite overdue for many more, but I also feel so enlivened, balanced, and nourished by the many I have received from my vibe. I'm curious to know your opinion. Do you believe vibrators to be valuable to a woman's pleasure?

— *Like My Vibe*

Dear Like My Vibe,

As we told Sneezeophiliac, we do not perform amputations. You can continue with your vibrator. That being said, if you are to become a serious student of sensuality your vibrator will have to be replaced by your hand, someone else's hand, and additionally a water-hose attachment. The vibrator is great if you want to use it to relieve tension with a short blast; however, it often numbs the nervous system, making it more difficult to receive lighter, more finessed touches. Perhaps you can wean yourself off it by doing exercises from our books and then only occasionally using it for old-time's sake.

If you wish to study with us we would ask you to put the old thing in mothballs and actively participate in your own training. You could always bring it back into use after you've finished with your training, though we doubt you would want to at that point.

My questions surround antidepressants and sexual desire. I have long suffered from severe depressive episodes, and, thankfully, with the grace and love of the divine, I feel back in the game again. I have such a devoted, adorable, loving, and supportive fiancé. He's seven years younger than me and has a very active sex drive. We have been together for five and a half years, and in the beginning our sex life was very *hot*. I love, adore, and cherish him, but sometimes I just don't desire sex, and I feel like there is something wrong with me. Although he acknowledges the fact that my libido may be low because of the meds I take, he also wonders if he just doesn't have it like he used to. He desires to adore me and give me pleasure, but sometimes I'm just not in the mood. In fact, I'm more not in the mood than in. Any thoughts on how I can spice up our sex life again?

— Wanting More

 Dear Wanting More,

Thank you for asking. You can have pleasure if you decide to. Your libido is part of you, but you are the one who has the final say. You are the decider of your desires. Read what we wrote to Libidoless Mom. You are in a similar place, and so are many women. Set aside some specific time and make it a priority to have some form of a sensual experience with your guy. You can do different things each time. For ideas, you can use some of the exercises in *To Bed or Not to Bed*. And don't forget to stimulate other parts of your bodies besides the genitals. Make it a fun game, not something you will want to avoid. Watch each other masturbate; think up fantasies that you and your partner will enjoy. Be creative, and don't wait for the libido fairy. Take a class in learning how to expand your orgasm and how to control one in someone else's body.

 Could you give us some information about the G-spot orgasm?

— Ms. Gee

Dear Ms Gee,

The term G-spot was coined in 1950 by Dr. Ernest Gräfenburg. Whether he found it on his wife or in the laboratory we are not sure. It refers to the spongy tissue in the front of the vaginal wall. The surface of the vaginal wall itself lacks specific nerve receptors for pressure, but the nerves that innervate the clitoris run through this area. These are the nerves that are stimulated when stroking the G-spot region.

Imagine the vaginal entry as a clock, with twelve o'clock at the top of the opening and six o'clock at the bottom, where it meets the perineum. The G-spot area would be found just inside the vagina, on the twelve o'clock side. If using two fingers, slightly spread them to avoid stimulating the exact center, which is where the urethral canal is located. Stimulation in this area can be painful to some women. On the other hand, some women actually enjoy being stroked here, so check things out and experiment. Position the hand palm up, with the pads of the index and middle fingers penetrating about one and a half to two inches inside the vagina, about up to the second knuckle. Stroke the spongy, bulbous tissue on the roof of the vagina with a come-hither motion.

Sometimes you can place the two fingers deeper inside the vagina and then crook them, pressing the back of the fingers against the top of the vagina to stimulate the G-spot. In either case, continue stimulating the head of the clitoris while you stimulate the G-spot. The head of the clitoris is where the highest concentration of nerve receptors is found, and the G-spot is one of the few areas inside the vagina that can be fun to stimulate after the head of the clitoris is engorged and orgasming. In our DEMO class we stimulate only the head of the clitoris for the first thirty minutes; then we penetrate with our fingers and include stimulation of the G-spot region. It can be a lot of fun to stroke these two areas simultaneously.

The G-spot is highly overhyped and was actually originally promoted in order to sell certain dildos or vibrators.

You wrote in your last message to me that just because my man does not want to do a session, it doesn't mean that *I* can't. Hmm. I'm not sure how to navigate that one. We're married, and, um, well, having someone else rub on my clit, even for training purposes—I don't think it would fly. If you recall, in the session we had with you, you coached him through it. Steve did not touch me.

That session with you changed my body forever. It awakened pleasure that I am still very much enjoying. I can only imagine what regular sessions would do to me. I want more. And, yes, there is a part of me that feels that it is my body and my right to awaken more—a part that is annoyed that I have to tiptoe around him. How have other students of yours successfully navigated this issue? Do you have any advice for me?

— *Wanting More*

 Dear Wanting More,

Now this is a fine question. It is one that a number of women face in more ways than just this specific scenario. For example, is it okay for a man other than your husband or boyfriend to buy you presents and to want to give you things? Is it okay to flirt with other men?

Many women who come to us have husbands who understand what we do and who do not feel threatened by it. They want their wives to have all the goodies that are available because they understand that having them will make their wives more fun, more appreciative, and kinder to them.

For the guys who resist this, it is usually about their egos. They think that because we are such experts they will compare unfavorably. This is not true. In fact, they will benefit from the opening up and blossoming of their beloved. It is their conditioning that gives them this narrow viewpoint. The issue is really about the state of your relationship and exactly how you want it to be, with both of you winning and getting what you each want. This is not only possible; it is really the only way to build the highest bond and intimacy that is achievable between two people. You do not want to have to "tiptoe"; you want to be able to speak and do as you see fit. You do not want to hurt him. You want him to want what you want. You want him to trust that your feelings are inclusive and beneficial to both of you.

So how, then, does a woman go about getting her guy to see the value of her goals? First of all, she must continue being nice. Getting angry at him won't help. Remember that it is the viewpoints that are getting in the way—not him. People think they are their viewpoints. But actually we are viewpoint holders. We can have multiple viewpoints, even on a single topic.

One way to cause a man to win, especially when he thinks he is going to lose, is to put him at cause for the goodies in your life, including the expansion of your orgasmic potential. That is, embrace a viewpoint that makes him a co-creator in this pleasure adventure, and communicate your appreciation to him regularly. Include him in what is happening with your goals and ideas; ask him for his input on how to get the things you want. Approach this as part of a team, and communicate better and more often in all areas of the relationship.

With regard to coming to see us for training sessions and workshops, some men may have other issues, such as the cost, or not wanting to have their beloved leave them for a few days, or whatever. Again, these issues can be negotiated and turned into a way for everybody to win.

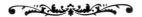

Bibliography

Alson, Sheila, and Gayle B. Burnett. *Peace in Everyday Relationships*. Alameda, CA: Hunter House Publishers, 2003.

Angier, Natalie. *Woman: An Intimate Geography*. New York: Houghton Mifflin, 1999.

Baranco, Vic. *Things I've Heard Vic Say,* vol. 6. Lafayette, CA: More University Press, 1991.

Bodansky, Steve and Vera. *To Bed or Not to Bed: What Men Want, What Women Want, How Great Sex Happens*. Alameda, CA: Hunter House Publishers, 2006.

Bodansky, Steve and Vera. *The Illustrated Guide to Extended Massive Orgasm*. Alameda, CA: Hunter House Publishers, 2002.

Bodansky, Steve and Vera. *Extended Massive Orgasm: How You Can Give and Receive Intense Sexual Pleasure*. Alameda, CA: Hunter House Publishers, 2000.

Chopra, Deepak. *Life after Death: The Burden of Proof*. New York: Harmony Books, Crown Publishers, 2006.

Davies, Clair, and Amber Davies. *The Trigger Point Therapy Workbook: Your Self-Treatment Guide for Pain Relief*. Oakland, CA: New Harbinger Publications, Inc., 2004.

Dawkins, Richard. *The Selfish Gene*. Oxford, UK: Oxford University Press, 1976.

Fisher, Helen. *The Sex Contract: The Evolution of Human Behavior*. New York: William Morrow, 1982.

Hofstadter, Douglas. *I Am a Strange Loop*. New York: Basic Books, 2007.

Kinsey, Alfred, Paul H. Gebhard, Clyde E. Martin, and Wardell B. Pomeroy. *Sexual Behavior in the Human Female*. Philadelphia, PA: W.B. Saunders Company, 1953.

Kundera, Milan. *Slowness*. New York: Harper Collins, 1995.

Masters, William H., Virginia E. Johnson, and Robert C. Kolodny. *Sex and Human Loving*. Boston, MA: Little, Brown and Co., 1982.

Minsky, Marvin. *The Society of Mind*. New York: Simon and Schuster, 1986.

Northrup, Christiane. *Women's Bodies, Women's Wisdom: Creating Physical and Emotional Health and Healing*. New York: Bantam, 2006.

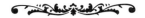

Index

Books on Orgasm, Seduction, and the G-Spot

EXTENDED MASSIVE ORGASM:
How You Can Give and Receive Intense Sexual Pleasure *by Steve Bodansky, PhD, & Vera Bodansky, PhD*

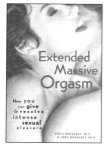

Yes, extended massive orgasms can be achieved! In this hands-on guide to doing it, Steve and Vera Bodansky describe how to take the experience of sex to a whole new level. Based on their research and work with clients, they explain the nature of orgasm, detailed techniques and positions for extended orgasm, and how partners can help each other overcome resistance to pleasure.

The authors disclose stimulation techniques and uniquely sensitive areas known only to specialized researchers, recommend the best positions for orgasm, and offer strategic advice for every technique from seduction to kissing. With the help of this book you'll find it's never too late — or too early — to make your partner ecstatic in the bedroom.

224 pages ... 5 illus. : 16 photos ... Paperback $14.95

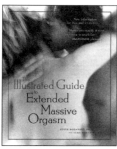

THE ILLUSTRATED GUIDE TO EXTENDED MASSIVE ORGASM
by Steve Bodansky, PhD, & Vera Bodansky, PhD

In this companion book, Steve and Vera Bodansky give much more detail about the best hand and body positions for performing and receiving EMO. More than 70 photographs and drawings illustrate genital anatomy and stimulation techniques, and the book covers new ground in the area of male arousal and orgasm.

Suddenly orgasm is no longer just a fleeting moment, but the beginning of lasting arousal that goes far beyond the bedroom.

256 pages ... 57 illus. : 25 photos ... Paperback $17.95

TO BED OR NOT TO BED:
What Men Want, What Women Want, How Great Sex Happens *by Vera Bodansky, PhD, & Steve Bodansky, PhD*

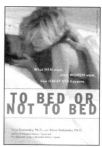

This saucy guide to seduction, better sex, and a great relationship was written by the Bodanskys to help both men and women get it on. In their extensive practice with clients, the authors have found that most men do not know what to do to get a woman to bed, or what to do when they get her there.

Women also want to have sex, but they have learned to put up obstacles for men so as not to be considered "easy." This book describes, with examples and exercises, what people can do to make getting into bed and having great sex possible, easier, and a whole lot of fun.

240 pages ... 12 illus. ... Paperback $14.95

FEMALE EJACULATION & THE G-SPOT
by Deborah Sundahl ... Forewords by Annie Sprinkle and Alice Ladas

Discover the G-spot's hidden sensations of intense pleasure. The G-spot is a woman's prostate gland. When stimulated, it swells with blood and emits ejaculate fluid, usually during orgasm. All women have a G-spot, and all women can ejaculate. Author Deborah

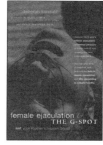

Sundahl has led seminars on female ejaculation for over 20 years, and her book delivers her research and exercises. Contents include techniques and positions that help a woman ejaculate and how men can help their female partners to ejaculate. Massage techniques developed by body-work specialists and Tantric healers are included along with exercises to help release emotional pain.

240 pages ... 13 illus. ... Paperback $16.95

Books on Sexual Pleasure, Healing, and Tantra

SEXUAL PLEASURE: Reaching New Heights of Sexual Arousal and Intimacy
by Barbara Keesling, PhD ... 2nd Edition

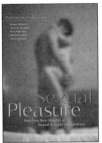

To experience deep sexual pleasure, Dr. Keesling explains, you must explore your ability to enjoy basic human touch. Focusing on touch and desire leads to greater passion, sensitivity, and fulfillment for both partners. Now Dr. Keesling has updated her classic bestseller after ten years, adding a new chapter on oral sex and 20 exercises never published before. There is material about talking sexy, the unique pleasures of different sexual positions, and choosing contraceptives based on pleasure. Written for couples and singles, this book is for everyone who wishes to give and receive deep, satisfying sexual pleasure.

264 pages ... 11 illus. : 16 photos ... Paperback $14.95

SEXUAL HEALING: The Completest Guide to Overcoming Common Sexual Problems
by Barbara Keesling, PhD ... 3rd Edition

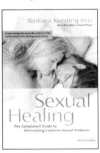

In this new edition of a classic, Barbara Keesling has combined material from the first two editions with new research and updates to create a definitive work in the field of sexual self-help.

The book offers more than 125 exercises to help treat a wide range of sexual problems, including premature ejaculation, low sexual desire, sexual anxiety, and sexual pain. It also describes using sexuality to heal your body, your feelings, and your relationship. The exercises can be used by people of any sexual orientation, and many exercises are helpful for older people. Sex therapists and psychotherapists will also find this book an invaluable resource for discussion and work with clients.

400 pages ... 4 illus. ... Paperback $18.95

MAKING LOVE BETTER THAN EVER: Reaching New Heights of Passion and Pleasure After 40 *by Barbara Keesling, PhD*

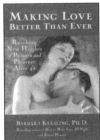

Great sex is not reserved for those under 40. With maturity comes the potential for a multi-faceted loving that draws from all we are and deepens our ties. This is the loving that sustains relationships into later years.

In this sensitive book, Dr. Keesling shows couples how to reignite sexual feelings and reconnect emotionally. She provides body-image and caress exercises that heighten sexual response and expand sexual potential, build self-esteem, open the lines of communication, and promote playfulness, spontaneity, and joy.

208 pages ... 6 photos ... Paperback $13.95

TANTRIC SEX FOR WOMEN: A Guide for Lesbian, Bi, Hetero and Solo Lovers
by Christa Schulte

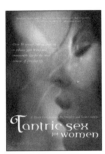

Every woman can enhance her sexual energy and add pleasure through the use of tantric ideas and exercises. Christa Schulte, a longtime practitioner of tantric methods, introduces women to *Tara-Tantra,* a woman-centered approach to sexuality and spirituality that she developed and has taught for many years.

Over 50 exercises and games form the heart of the book ... for solo-lovers, love games for two, rituals, meditations, and massage techniques, all designed to enable women of every sexual orientation to explore their sexual and sensual potential, enrich their relationships, and enjoy the small ecstasies of everyday life. The book will also help men who want to understand women's sexuality better and become deeper, more fulfilling partners.

288 pages ... 3 illus. : 15 photos ... Paperback $16.95